THE 30-DAY HORMONE SOLUTION

The Key to **BETTER HEALTH** and

Natural Weight Loss

SAMANTHA GLADISH,
Weight Loss and Women's Hormone Coach

PAGE STREET
PUBLISHING CO.

PAGE STREET
PUBLISHING CO.

First published in 2019 by
Page Street Publishing Co.
27 Congress Street, Suite 105
Salem, MA 01970
www.pagestreetpublishing.com

Distributed by Macmillan, sales in Canada by The Canadian Manda Group.

23 22 21 20 19   1 2 3 4 5

ISBN-13: 978-1-62414-991-7
ISBN-10: 1-62414-991-X

Library of Congress Control Number: 2019940367

Cover and book design by Meg Baskis for Page Street Publishing Co.
Lifestyle photography by Nat Caron Photography, Food photography by Trish Hughes
Infographics by Vanessa Fioretti

Printed and bound in China

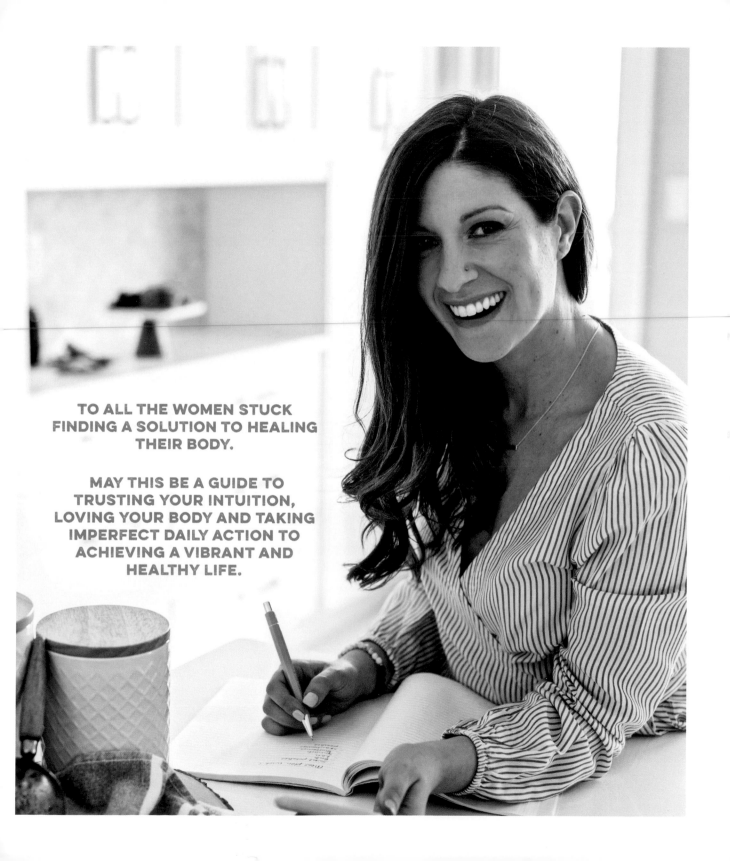

TO ALL THE WOMEN STUCK
FINDING A SOLUTION TO HEALING
THEIR BODY.

MAY THIS BE A GUIDE TO
TRUSTING YOUR INTUITION,
LOVING YOUR BODY AND TAKING
IMPERFECT DAILY ACTION TO
ACHIEVING A VIBRANT AND
HEALTHY LIFE.

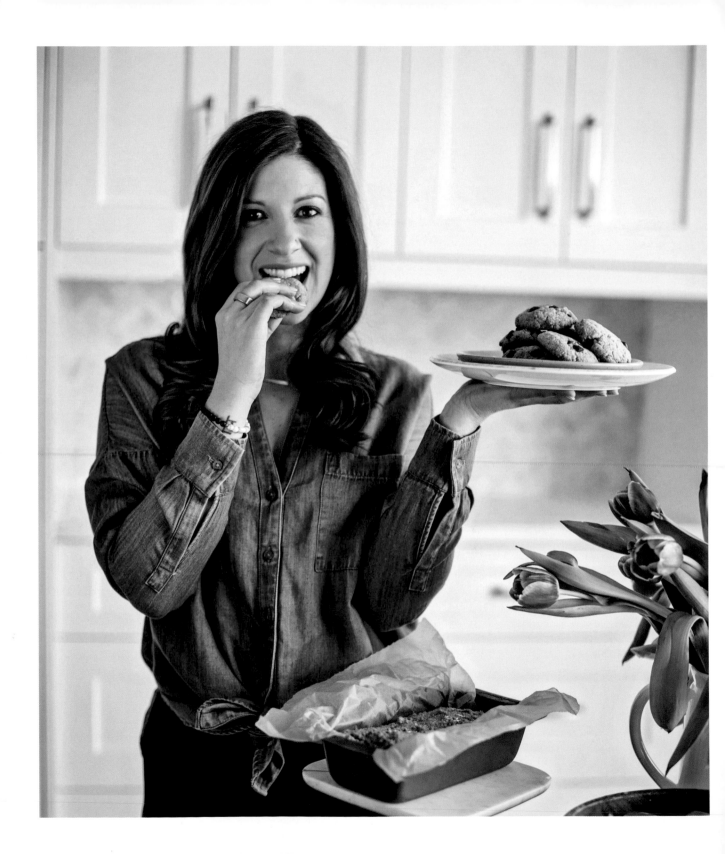

CONTENTS

WHY THE 30-DAY HORMONE SOLUTION IS DIFFERENT

Welcome! I bet that you're here because you're looking for answers to heal your thyroid, support your menstrual cycle, lose weight and just feel better. When it comes to our health, we all want something different. But universally, it's safe to say that we all want to feel and look good.

As with many health practitioners, I started in this industry because of my own health crisis, looking for answers and help. I want to share my own personal story with you, because I've been in the trenches, just as you are. I want you to know that there is a better way and there is a solution.

My journey started when I was a little girl. I was always innately interested in food and nutrition, and I spent so much time outdoors and in the garden. In fact, I remember my parents taking me to McDonald's and I would order salad. Yes—true story! That's not to say I never had any Big Macs, because I've had plenty of those. But I was always connected in some way to healthy food.

I was also lucky enough to grow up in a household where my mother made everything from scratch and would literally cringe at packaged foods. But—as most teenagers tend to do—I ate lots of carbs and sugary foods. My idea of healthy food back in the day was margarine, low-fat foods, whole-wheat anything and artificial low-calorie sweeteners.

I struggled with terrible PMS as a teenager that left me in bed curled up for days. Because of this, I went on the birth control pill, not truly understanding the effects it was having on my ovulation and hormones. I remember being in my doctor's office telling him how bad my period pain was. I also thought to myself, "Well, if all my friends are on the pill, then I should be too!"

Without any hesitation, my doctor handed me a pack of pills and I started on them that very day. In fact, I continued taking them for seven years.

I also struggled with migraines, headaches and terrible digestion. My gut health took quite the hit over the years—from over-the-counter meds, antibiotics if I got sick, the birth control pill. . . . Oh, and I can't forget the parasite I caught on vacation in my mid-twenties, which led to antiparasitics, antifungals and more gut damage.

Fast-forward to my university years: I was working out regularly, in great shape, lean, energetic and eating really well. But all of this was coupled with some very late nights of studying and partying, along with drinking and late-night fast food. I remember how bloated I would get after eating and how bad my migraines would get at times—leaving me to go to bed, turn off all the lights, drown out all sound and just lie there until it all went away.

During my university years, I dated a guy whose family was into organic food, homeopathics and nutrition. It sparked a huge interest for me! I loved learning about food and how it affected our bodies and how you could use all-natural remedies to heal and support your health. This led me to enroll in the Canadian School of Natural Nutrition, where I studied to become a holistic nutritionist. From there I went on to take courses in immunology, cancer care, homeopathics, hormones and functional nutrition.

Fitness was also a huge part of my life. As a kid, I spent a lot of time outdoors and playing sports. From soccer to basketball to gymnastics, I was a very active young girl. As I got older, I found a love for weight lifting, which led me to become a certified personal trainer. I also taught kickboxing and Pilates classes, and I even received my 200-hour yoga teacher training certificate.

I remember my first week at nutrition school. I sat at the front of the class, and it was as though a light bulb had gone off. In that very first week I learned how detrimental the birth control pill was, how it was robbing my body of essential nutrients and impairing my gut health. In that moment, I stopped taking it, started to ditch the fake "diet" foods (aka margarine, artificial sweeteners and low-fat foods) and got on a hormone-balancing post-pill supplement protocol. I cared for my body and health like never before.

This passion led me to want to help other women to support their hormones and bodies with whole food nutrition, strategic supplementation and lifestyle interventions. But it didn't end there.

Fast-forward to early 2017: I was a busy entrepreneur working hard on growing and building my online nutrition business when I started to feel off. I was extremely tired, and I felt puffy and achy. I had gained a couple of extra pounds. I couldn't sleep, and I started experiencing painful aches and pains in my hands, fingers and wrists. At this point, I had coached hundreds of women in my practice and these symptoms, although new to me, were something I was quite familiar with from working with my clients.

One day while working out, I had a hard time gripping and holding my weights. The pain in my hands was unbearable. In that instant I said to myself, "This is Hashimoto's thyroiditis."

A few weeks later I went to my naturopath and got a requisition for a full thyroid panel. Conventional medicine only tests for thyroid stimulating hormone or TSH—something we'll dive into in Chapter 3 (page 27). I knew I needed a full panel to truly get a clear picture of what was going on with my thyroid and test for autoimmune antibodies.

Sure enough, my labs confirmed I had Hashimoto's and my antibodies were quite high. This confirmation led me down the path of deeper healing. I started on the Autoimmune Paleo Protocol (AIP) diet, revamped my supplement regime and made sleep my top priority. Within weeks I had already started to feel a difference, and within six months my antibodies had dropped by half.

Autoimmunity runs in my family. There is often a genetic disposition, along with gut dysbiosis and environmental triggers that can affect autoimmune function. It's safe to say that all those years of antibiotics, over-the-counter meds and the pill definitely played a role in my autoimmune diagnosis.

My diet has drastically changed over the years, and where I am today with my health has been a twenty-plus-year journey of experimenting, learning and testing. Wherever you are with your journey, this is the perfect starting point to dive in, be open, experiment, learn and test for yourself.

If there's one thing I know for sure, it's that when women start to take care of themselves and fuel their bodies with nutrition, movement and a whole lot of self-love and kindness, they start to stand more powerfully, make better choices and create more possibilities for their lives. And I know this to be true from my own personal experience with health and hormones, as well as the experiences of thousands of women I've coached over the years.

When it comes to supporting our health and hormones, there are many areas that we need to start focusing on—nutrition, sleep, stress management, detoxification, exercise, beauty care, environment, relationships and so much more. We'll explore many of these topics thoroughly in this book. Having more of these health pieces in place means we enjoy a better quality of life, less disease, more vitality and better hormonal health.

Healing is a journey. And if there is ONE thing I can say to you about your health, it's this: *You need to start paying attention to the whispers of your body. You need to listen—closely.* If you feel something is off with your body, don't ignore it. Don't just think your symptoms are normal because "you're getting older." It is time to TUNE INTO *your body and know that it's never too late for transformation.*

The 30-Day Hormone Solution will guide you through the strategies and tools I use in my private practice with clients to help them shed weight and balance their hormones. My 30-day program explains exactly what to eat and when to eat, and it provides you with the important reset rules to help you achieve incredible weight loss and hormone success.

If you've been following me on Instagram @holisticwellnessfoodie or my website at www .holisticwellness.ca, you know that when it comes to food, I don't disappoint. Losing weight and balancing hormones doesn't need to be bland and boring. The recipes in this book are delicious and easy to make, and they will help reduce bloating, detox excess estrogen, support your thyroid, improve gut health and shed those extra pounds!

This reset has been the difference and the "aha moment" for hundreds of women, helping them *finally* lose fat and feel better. It uses the principles of how food actually affects fat loss so that you aren't blindly restricting food, making yourself miserable and setting yourself up to fail again. Spoiler alert: It's hormones, not calories, that call the shots.

I'd love for you to enjoy a program that turns into a lifestyle—one that's delicious, nourishing and totally revitalizing. And one that helps you shed the pounds and turn back the aging clock! And that's exactly what you'll get with *The 30-Day Hormone Solution*. I thought to myself: "If I only had 30 days to work with you, to help you improve your health and hormones, what would I do? What strategies would I implement? What nutrition and supplement protocols would help move the needle the most?"

And that is how this book was born. It will help you achieve incredible hormonal health in 30 days using simple, effective and delicious protocols.

I hope this book becomes the inspiration and education you need to create lasting change with your health, your hormones and your life.

Samantha Gladish

PART 1:

UNDER-STANDING HORMONAL BALANCE

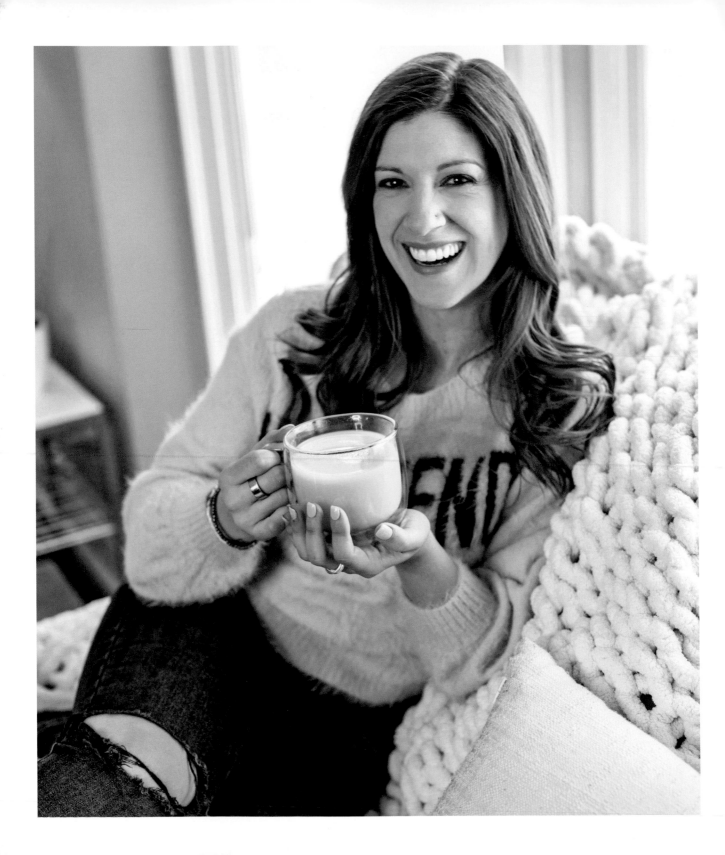

CHAPTER 1:

HORMONES 101

Your hormones dictate a lot about your health—from digestion to weight, brain health, energy, mood, memory, sex drive, sleep and fertility. Your hormones are involved in a very delicate balance. When one becomes imbalanced, it creates a cascade effect, affecting other hormones in the body and causing more imbalances. Hormonal imbalances do not exist in isolation, and this is why there is no "one simple fix." It's all interconnected.

In my practice, the top hormones I see out of balance with women are cortisol, thyroid, estrogen and insulin. These hormones affect the brain, mood, stress levels and weight. When we're under acute stress, cortisol is our main fuel for focus, attention and function. However, chronic stress can lead to cortisol levels that are too high, which can often lead to levels that are too low over time. Hello burnout! Cortisol also governs our blood sugar, blood pressure and immune function. Ever find you catch a cold or a flu or you feel completely depleted during a high-stress time? That's because there is a direct correlation between decreased immune function and high cortisol levels.

Our thyroid affects our metabolism and our mood, menstrual cycle, energy, sleep, digestion and weight. It also governs the metabolism of the ovaries, and it is a key player for fertility. When our thyroid is in balance, we feel energetic, sexy and happy, and we sleep deeply. We'll be looking at cortisol and the thyroid in more depth in Chapter 3, page 27.

As for estrogen, I like to refer to this hormone as the "sex kitten." Estrogen helps keep us lubricated, juicy, feminine, in flow and energetic. It also works to regulate menstruation by building up the uterine lining to help us prepare for pregnancy. Estradiol, the queen bee of estrogens, helps boost neurotransmitters such as serotonin and dopamine, which is why it has a dramatic effect on our happy moods. We'll be looking at estrogen in more depth in Chapter 2, page 17.

Insulin is our blood sugar regulator and directs our muscles, liver and fat cells to take up glucose from the blood and store it. If you're eating high-sugar foods—and even fruits—you'll get a big spike in blood sugar. Your pancreas then has to produce insulin in an effort to move that sugar into your cells. But here's the kicker: When insulin levels go up, so does cortisol, the stress hormone. Cortisol competes with progesterone for the same receptors. Unfortunately, cortisol always wins this fight. Hello, low progesterone! So, progesterone often goes down, eventually leaving you in a state of progesterone deficiency or estrogen dominance—think PMS, polycystic ovary syndrome (PCOS), endometriosis, fibroids, heavy and painful periods, migraines, depression, anxiety, acne . . . and the list goes on. Can you see what I mean by our hormones being interconnected? We'll be looking at insulin in more depth in Chapter 4, page 41.

In addition to cortisol, thyroid, estrogen and insulin, there are many hormones that affect our health and body. Progesterone counterbalances estrogen, and it is what I like to refer to as the "fat cat." I like to think of it as the hormone that wants to cuddle up on the couch with a blanket like your cat would and indulge in a delicious piece of chocolate. With that said, it *won't* make you fat; in fact, it will *help* your body burn fat, when it is in balance. Progesterone is the hormone that helps us slow down, sleep well and feel balanced. It also helps keep our moods stable and regulates the uterine lining.

Testosterone is often referred to as the "man's hormone," and although men produce more testosterone than women, we do produce a small amount of it, which can help with our sex drive, vitality and bone and brain health. In women with PCOS, we often see higher levels of testosterone, leading to symptoms of facial hair growth or cystic acne.

Leptin and ghrelin are our hunger hormones. Leptin controls hunger and plays a role in fat gain and fat loss, determining whether or not we will use food as fuel or store it. Leptin decreases hunger, while ghrelin increases hunger. I like to think of ghrelin as the "gremlin hormone," always on the lookout for more food. Your stomach makes ghrelin when it's empty. Just like leptin, ghrelin goes into the blood, crosses the blood-brain barrier and ends up at your hypothalamus, where it tells your brain, "Hey, I'm hungry!" Both hormones regulate appetite and hunger, and both of them regulate homeostasis, keeping things stable and balanced in the body.

Take the hormone questionnaire (on pages 14–15) to help determine which of your hormones might be out of balance.

REAL TALK

Before you dive into the questionnaire, let's have a quick chat about good ol' doctor Google. You know what I mean—you feel like you have every symptom under the sun and then go on Google to research it, and sure enough you've diagnosed yourself with some very rare disease and start to freak out. We've all done it. Don't get me wrong: the Internet can be very helpful, but what I really want you to gain from filling out the questionnaire that follows is awareness. Awareness that something is off in your body and it's time to dive in and put some healing practices in place, which is exactly why this book is in your hands. When I first started on my path of healing my body and hormones, I was overwhelmed. But step by step, I started to introduce new foods and supplements, found workouts that excited me and removed foods from my diet that no longer made me feel energized and only depleted me. It was a process, and it started with baby steps. So wherever you are on your journey and whatever the questionnaire might reveal for you, it all boils down to the same thing: making a choice to create change and step into a more powerful version of yourself. And the good news is that the recipes and the meal plan in this book will help you do just that!

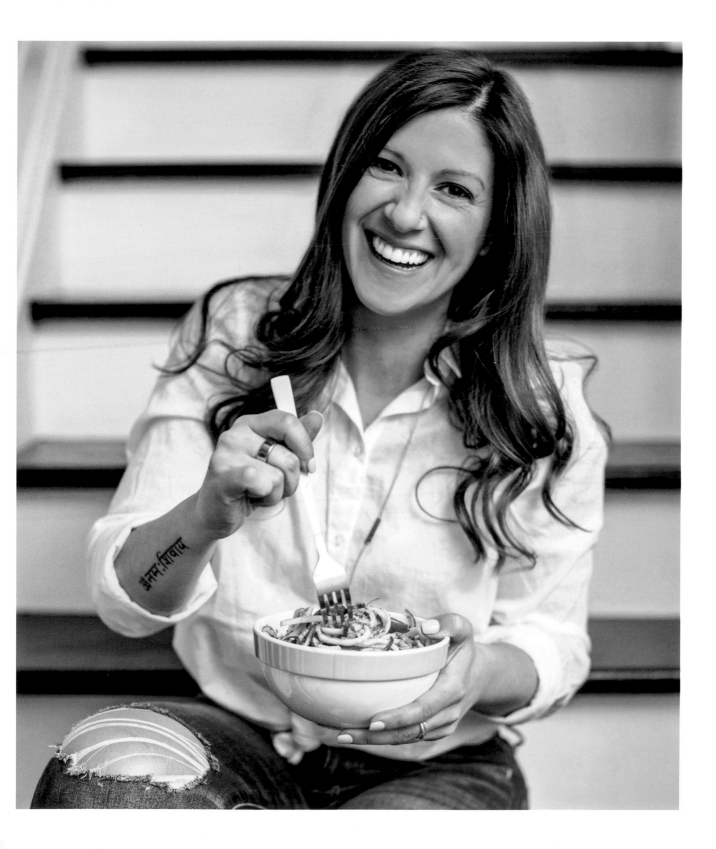

HEALTHY HORMONE QUESTIONNAIRE FOR WOMEN

CHECK ALL THAT APPLY.

SECTION A

- ☐ RACING FROM ONE ACTIVITY TO ANOTHER, OR FEELING LIKE YOU ARE
- ☐ FEELING TIRED YET UNABLE TO RELAX OR SLEEP
- ☐ FEELING NERVOUS OR JITTERY
- ☐ INABILITY TO CALM DOWN AT NIGHT BEFORE BEDTIME
- ☐ GETTING A SECOND WIND LATE AT NIGHT
- ☐ DIFFICULTY FALLING ASLEEP
- ☐ A FEELING OF ANXIETY
- ☐ IRRITABLE BOWEL SYNDROME (IBS)
- ☐ WORRYING ABOUT THINGS, EVEN THOSE YOU CANNOT CONTROL
- ☑ ANGER ISSUES—FINDING YOURSELF YELLING OR SNAPPING
- ☐ MEMORY ISSUES AND INABILITY TO FOCUS
- ☑ SUGAR CRAVINGS, INCLUDING WANTING SOMETHING SWEET AFTER MEALS
- ☑ WEIGHT GAIN AROUND THE MIDDLE, NOT RELATED TO BLOATING
- ☐ ECZEMA AND THINNING OF THE SKIN
- ☐ BONE LOSS
- ☐ RAPID HEART BEAT AND/OR HIGH BLOOD PRESSURE
- ☐ HIGH BLOOD SUGAR AND POSSIBLE INSULIN RESISTANCE AND DIABETES
- ☐ FEELINGS OF WEAKNESS OR SHAKINESS BETWEEN MEALS
- ☐ HEADACHES, ESPECIALLY IF A MEAL IS MISSED
- ☐ SLOWER RECOVERY FROM A PHYSICAL INJURY THAN IN THE PAST
- ☐ PINKISH PURPLE STRETCH MARKS ON BELLY OR BACK (NOT RELATED TO PREGNANCY)
- ☑ MENSTRUAL CYCLES ARE NOT REGULAR
- ☐ FERTILITY ISSUES

SECTION C

- ☐ FEELING AGITATED
- ☐ PMS
- ☐ HEADACHES THAT OCCUR AT REGULAR TIMES DURING YOUR CYCLE, INCLUDING HORMONAL MIGRAINES
- ☑ SORE AND/OR SWOLLEN BREASTS
- ☐ WEIGHT GAIN
- ☐ MOOD SWINGS, ANXIETY AND/OR DEPRESSION
- ☐ MENSTRUAL CYCLES ARE IRREGULAR MAYBE EVEN BECOMING MORE FREQUENT
- ☐ HEAVY, PAINFUL PERIODS
- ☐ GAINING 3–5 POUNDS BEFORE YOUR PERIOD
- ☐ SIGNS OF FLUID RETENTION SUCH AS BLOATING AROUND THE BELLY OR PUFFY ANKLES
- ☐ OVARIAN CYSTS, FIBROCYSTIC BREASTS OR ENDOMETRIAL CYSTS OR POLYPS
- ☐ DISRUPTED SLEEP
- ☐ RESTLESS OR ITCHY LEGS, ESPECIALLY AT NIGHT
- ☐ POOR COORDINATION
- ☐ CONSTIPATION
- ☐ INFERTILITY OR DIFFICULTY GETTING PREGNANT
- ☐ MISCARRIAGE IN THE FIRST TRIMESTER
- ☐ THYROID ISSUES
- ☐ HOT FLASHES
- ☐ INCREASED INTESTINAL ISSUES

SECTION B

- ☐ USING CAFFEINE TO GIVE YOU ENERGY EITHER IN THE MORNING OR THROUGHOUT THE DAY
- ☐ FALLING ASLEEP WHILE READING OR WATCHING TV
- ☐ FEELING FATIGUED OR BURNED OUT
- ☐ LOSS OF STAMINA, ESPECIALLY IN THE MIDAFTERNOON
- ☐ FEELING CYNICAL OR HAVING A NEGATIVE PERSPECTIVE
- ☐ CRYING FOR NO PARTICULAR REASON
- ☐ LOWER ABILITY TO PROBLEM-SOLVE
- ☐ EVERYTHING SEEMS HARDER TO DO THAN IT USED TO BE
- ☐ FEELING STRESSED AND HAVING TROUBLE COPING WITH IT
- ☐ LESS ABILITY TO HANDLE STRESS
- ☐ INABILITY TO FALL ASLEEP AND STAY ASLEEP—MAY WAKE UP AT 3:00 OR 4:00 IN THE MORNING AND NOT BE ABLE TO GET BACK TO SLEEP
- ☐ LOW BLOOD PRESSURE
- ☑ STANDING UP QUICKLY AND FEELING DIZZY
- ☐ DIFFICULTY FIGHTING FLUS AND COLDS OR HEALING WOUNDS
- ☐ ISSUES WITH ASTHMA, ALLERGIES OR BRONCHITIS
- ☐ BLOOD SUGAR FLUCTUATIONS THROUGHOUT THE DAY
- ☐ CRAVINGS FOR SALT
- ☐ EXCESS SWEATING
- ☐ FEELINGS OF NAUSEA; VOMITING OR LOOSE STOOLS
- ☐ ALTERNATING DIARRHEA AND CONSTIPATION
- ☐ MUSCLE WEAKNESS, ESPECIALLY AROUND THE JOINTS LIKE KNEES AND ELBOWS
- ☐ MUSCLE AND/OR JOINT PAIN
- ☐ HEMORRHOIDS AND/OR VARICOSE VEINS
- ☐ SKIN BRUISES EASILY
- ☐ SUDDEN HEART PALPITATIONS OR IRREGULAR HEARTBEAT

SECTION D

- ☐ SIGNS OF WATER RETENTION SUCH AS BLOATING AND PUFFINESS
- ☐ ABNORMAL PAP SMEARS
- ☑ HEAVY BLEEDING DURING PERIODS
- ☐ POST-MENOPAUSAL BLEEDING
- ☐ GAIN WEIGHT EASILY, PARTICULARLY IN THE HIPS AND BUTT
- ☐ BREAST SIZE INCREASE
- ☑ SWOLLEN BREASTS
- ☐ FIBROIDS
- ☐ ENDOMETRIOSIS OR PAINFUL PERIODS
- ☑ MOOD SWINGS, DEPRESSION OR FEELING IRRITABLE
- ☐ PMS
- ☐ TROUBLE SLEEPING
- ☐ MEMORY ISSUES
- ☐ COLD HANDS OR FEET
- ☐ HAIR LOSS

SECTION E

- ☑ MEMORY ISSUES, SUCH AS GOING TO GET SOMETHING AND FORGETTING WHAT IT WAS WHEN YOU GET THERE
- ☐ FEELING EMOTIONALLY FRAGILE IN COMPARISON TO HOW YOU FELT WHEN YOU WERE YOUNGER
- ☐ DEPRESSION, OFTEN COMBINED WITH ANXIETY OR LETHARGY
- ☐ AGING OF THE SKIN
- ☐ DRY SKIN AND EYES
- ☑ WEIGHT GAIN
- ☐ HOT FLASHES AND/OR NIGHT SWEATS
- ☐ SLEEP ISSUES, SUCH AS WAKING UP IN THE MIDDLE OF THE NIGHT
- ☐ VAGINAL DRYNESS
- ☐ LOSS OF LIBIDO
- ☐ ANXIETY
- ☐ MOOD SWINGS
- ☐ INABILITY TO FOCUS
- ☐ INTESTINAL INFLAMMATORY ISSUES

SECTION G

- ☐ HAIR LOSS OR HAIR THINNING, INCLUDING EYEBROWS AND EYELASHES
- ☐ DRY SKIN AND HAIR (EASILY TANGLES)
- ☐ THIN, BRITTLE FINGERNAILS
- ☐ FLUID RETENTION AND/OR PUFFY ANKLES
- ☑ GAINING WEIGHT AND DIFFICULTY LOSING WEIGHT
- ☐ HIGH CHOLESTEROL
- ☐ CONSTIPATION (BOWEL MOVEMENTS FEWER THAN ONCE A DAY)
- ☐ RECURRING HEADACHES
- ☐ DECREASED ABILITY TO SWEAT
- ☑ MUSCLE OR JOINT ACHES
- ☐ INABILITY TO MAINTAIN MUSCLE MASS
- ☐ TINGLING IN HANDS AND/OR FEET
- ☐ COLD HANDS AND FEET
- ☐ INTOLERANCE OR SENSITIVITY TO HEAT AND/OR COLD
- ☐ SLOW SPEECH OR HOARSENESS
- ☐ A SLOWER HEART RATE
- ☐ LETHARGY AND LACK OF ENERGY
- ☐ FATIGUE, PARTICULARLY IN THE MORNING
- ☑ DIFFICULTY CONCENTRATING AND FEELING LIKE YOUR BRAIN IS RUNNING SLOWER
- ☐ SLOWER REACTION TIME (REFLEXES ARE SLOWER)
- ☐ LOW SEX DRIVE FOR NO PARTICULAR REASON
- ☐ DEPRESSION OR MOOD SWINGS
- ☐ TAKING ANTIDEPRESSANTS BUT THEY ARE NOT WORKING
- ☑ HEAVY PERIODS OR OTHER MENSTRUAL ISSUES
- ☐ PREGNANCY ISSUES, SUCH AS INFERTILITY, MISCARRIAGE AND PERHAPS PREMATURE BIRTH
- ☐ AN ENLARGED THYROID (OR GOITER), SWOLLEN TONGUE
- ☐ DIFFICULTY SWALLOWING
- ☐ A FAMILY HISTORY OF THYROID PROBLEMS

SECTION F

- ☐ NEW FACIAL HAIR GROWTH AND/OR MORE HAIR ON ARMS AND CHEST
- ☐ ACNE
- ☐ GREASY HAIR AND/OR SKIN
- ☐ THINNING HAIR ON HEAD
- ☐ DARKER COLOR AND THICKER SKIN UNDER ARMPITS
- ☐ SKIN TAGS, ESPECIALLY ON THE NECK AND UPPER BODY
- ☐ LOW BLOOD SUGAR OR HIGH BLOOD SUGAR OR FLUCTUATIONS BETWEEN HIGH AND LOW THROUGH OUT THE DAY
- ☑ IRRITABILITY AND/OR AGGRESSIVE BEHAVIOR (PRONE TO ARGUMENTS AND FIGHTS)
- ☐ DEPRESSION, OFTEN ACCOMPANIED BY ANXIETY
- ☐ OVARIAN CYSTS
- ☐ MID-CYCLE PAIN
- ☐ INFERTILITY AND ISSUES WITH GETTING PREGNANT
- ☐ POLYCYSTIC OVARIAN SYNDROME (PCOS)
- ☐ DECREASED INTEREST IN SEX
- ☑ WEIGHT GAIN AND DIFFICULTY LOSING WEIGHT
- ☐ DIFFICULTY CONCENTRATING
- ☐ FATIGUE AND EXHAUSTION

SECTION H

- ☐ DISRUPTED SLEEP
- ☐ FATIGUE
- ☐ DIMINISHED INTEREST IN SEX
- ☑ WEIGHT GAIN
- ☐ DEPRESSION AND ANXIETY
- ☐ OSTEOPOROSIS
- ☐ HAIR LOSS
- ☐ INABILITY TO MAINTAIN MUSCLE MASS OR BUILD MUSCLE
- ☐ INABILITY TO HAVE ORGASMS
- ☐ DRY, THINNING SKIN
- ☐ DECREASED COGNITIVE FUNCTION
- ☐ INABILITY TO FOCUS AND CONCENTRATE
- ☑ IRREGULAR PERIODS
- ☐ DECREASED COLON FUNCTION AND POSSIBLE CONSTIPATION

SECTION I

- ☐ POLYCYSTIC OVARIAN SYNDROME (PCOS)
- ☐ PRONE TO BLOOD SUGAR HIGHS AND LOWS
- ☐ INCREASE IN INSULIN AND PRONE TO INSULIN RESISTANCE
- ☐ ACNE
- ☐ INCREASED HAIR LOSS
- ☐ INCREASED FACIAL AND BODY HAIR
- ☑ MOOD AND ANGER ISSUES

RESULTS: THREE OR MORE CHECKS IN ANY ONE SECTION MAY INDICATE THE HORMONE ISSUE ASSOCIATED WITH THAT SECTION. FIVE OR MORE CHECKS MAY WARRANT SEEING A PRACTITIONER TO GET YOUR HORMONES TESTED AND CHECK FOR OTHER HEALTH ISSUES. DON'T BE SURPRISED IF YOU HAVE ISSUES IN MORE THAN ONE SECTION, AS EACH HORMONE CAN AFFECT ANOTHER. SUPPORTING THE HEALTH OF ALL HORMONES WITH GOOD DIET AND LIFESTYLE CHOICES IS THE GOAL.

SECTION A: HIGH CORTISOL
SECTION B: LOW CORTISOL

SECTION C: LOW PROGESTERONE
SECTION D: HIGH ESTROGEN

SECTION E: LOW ESTROGEN
SECTION F: LOW ANDROGENS

SECTION G: LOW THYROID
SECTION H: LOW TESTOSTERONE
SECTION I: HIGH TESTOSTERONE

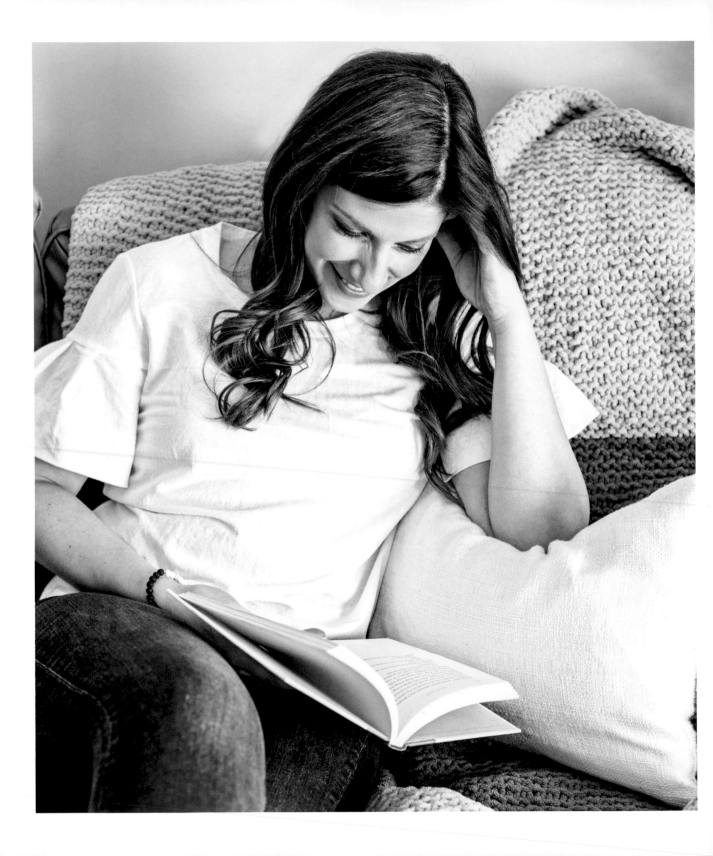

CHAPTER 2:

YOUR MONTHLY REPORT CARD:

YOUR MENSTRUAL CYCLE

Let's dive into the four phases of your cycle to see what's really going on and why you feel different week to week. I want you to think of your cycle and your period as your monthly report card. It can help you determine the *why* behind your symptoms.

Feel moody, exhausted, groggy and snappy just before your period? It could be low progesterone. Have heavy periods accompanied by water retention and breast tenderness? It could be high estrogen. Paying attention to these symptoms will help you become the best detective of your hormonal health, and no one knows your body better than you do, so tune in!

It's important to note that a regular cycle for you might be closer to 24 days or 35 days; 28 days is the average, but not the rule.

The chart on page 18 outlines your menstrual cycle. You can see the hormones that are working their magic, based on the phase of your cycle. It's important to note that each hormone requires the one that came before it for production— that's why it's called a cycle or a period, because it comes on periodically. Often, we hear that low progesterone could be the culprit to a lot of hormonal issues related to PMS. However, high levels of estrogen can throw off progesterone balance. Your hormones work in harmony, so when one is off, they will all generally be out of balance in some way or another.

PHASE 1: THE FOLLICULAR PHASE
DURATION: TYPICALLY 7 TO 10 DAYS

A healthy period begins with healthy follicles. Day 1 of your period—the first day you bleed—is marked by the follicular phase. I've broken up your cycle into four phases, keeping menstruation as its own phase, for some deeper insight into your cycle overall. Generally speaking, your period and the follicular phase are the same. During this phase, your hypothalamus will signal your pituitary gland to release follicular stimulating hormone (FSH), which is sent to your ovaries to prepare them for the release of an egg. Estrogen, testosterone and progesterone levels are all at their lowest at the beginning of this phase. As you near ovulation, your estrogen levels start to increase; this helps thicken the uterine lining and host an egg.

If you are estrogen dominant and suffer from any conditions related to an estrogen imbalance, you may experience more symptoms during this phase. At this time, it is key to consume foods that support the right amount of estrogen and work to support detoxification. Broccoli, cauliflower, cabbage and fermented foods, such as sauerkraut and kimchi, are good options.

FEMALE MENSTRUAL CHART
OVULATION PROCESS AND HORMONE LEVELS

DAYS*

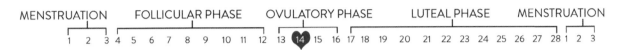

| MENSTRUATION | FOLLICULAR PHASE | OVULATORY PHASE | LUTEAL PHASE | MENSTRUATION |

1 2 3 4 5 6 7 8 9 10 11 12 13 14 15 16 17 18 19 20 21 22 23 24 25 26 27 28 1 2 3

*THIS IS BASED ON A 28-DAY CYCLE.
PLEASE NOTE DATES CAN VARY BASED ON LENGTH OF YOUR CYCLE.

HORMONE LEVEL

- LH
- FSH
- ESTROGEN
- PROGESTERONE

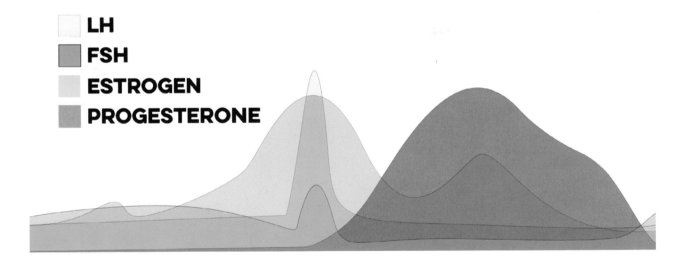

Toward the end of this phase, if your hormones are in balance, you will physically experience more energy and vitality. For those who tend to be more estrogen dominant, you may suffer from some anxiety and irritability. Generally, most women feel good physically and emotionally during this phase and can handle more strenuous activities and exercise.

PHASE 2: OVULATORY PHASE
DURATION: TYPICALLY 3 TO 4 DAYS

Ovulation is essentially the most important phase of your cycle and, in a way, the other three phases revolve around it. During this phase, you will experience a sharp rise in FSH followed by an increase in luteinizing hormone (LH). Thanks to a sharp increase in testosterone and estrogen, you experience more arousal and are most fertile during this time. Hello sexy time! An egg is also released into one of the fallopian tubes, and the uterine lining further thickens.

Women who are estrogen dominant or have reproductive issues may experience what is known as ovulation pain. It can last anywhere from a few hours to three to four days. The level of discomfort ranges from a slight twinge of pain to a consistent uncomfortable pain, especially in and around the ovaries. Excess estrogen can also increase bloating and acne at this time, and some women might find they are prone to migraines or headaches. Physically speaking, thanks to a rise in testosterone, this is a great time to work out. Swimming, running, spin class or weight training may feel easier to do at this time in your cycle. Also, don't be surprised if you feel especially attractive, as this is nature's way for you to attract a mate!

During ovulation, due to an increase in energy output, I encourage you to tune into your body and its cravings. Do you find you are being called to a plate of pasta? It is common to crave carbohydrates during this phase, so the best plan of action is to introduce more fibrous, starchier vegetables, such as plantains, skin-on sweet potatoes and squashes.

PHASE 3: LUTEAL PHASE
DURATION: TYPICALLY 10 TO 14 DAYS

The luteal phase generally causes the most concern for women. Progesterone starts to peak during this phase, which signals the body to keep the uterine lining intact. Both FSH and LH levels drop, which helps ensure that only one egg is released into the uterus. Estrogen levels continue to rise, and progesterone levels halt as this phase comes to an end, and that in turn triggers your period.

If your hormones are not in balance, PMS symptoms are going to occur. One of the key factors during this time is stress. Stress means the adrenal glands are producing too much cortisol. The cortisol interferes with progesterone production, and this creates estrogen dominance. Don't be surprised if your energy levels are at an all-time low too. Loading up on stress-supportive vitamins, such as vitamin C and B vitamins, is especially important during this phase. Also, magnesium will support liver detoxification, reduce period cramping and help you sleep more soundly.

It's essential to get the proper amount of sleep and to slow down during this phase. Due to decreasing energy levels, you might find exercise such as walking and yoga more pleasurable, and both work great to reduce stress. Most women tend to feel fatigued and start to experience symptoms such as bloating, irritability, cravings and mood swings just before heading into their period. Try practicing meditation, mindfulness or deep breathing techniques; all can be helpful, especially if you are feeling anxious or irritable.

PHASE 4: MENSTRUAL PHASE
DURATION: TYPICALLY 3 TO 7 DAYS

When the body has gone through the first three phases and fertilization has not occurred, it is time for the menstrual phase. Due to progesterone levels dropping, your uterine lining starts to shed and you start to menstruate, also known as your period or bleeding phase. Estrogen will peak and then drop, which stimulates your brain to prepare for another four-phase cycle.

During this time, there will be a combination of red and brown bleeding—although for the first few days of your cycle, your period should be bright red. Women often experience lower backaches, fatigue, cravings and cramps, although sometimes there is a sense of relief as your estrogen peak passes. Many women with hormonal issues endure severe cramping during this phase. To reduce the severity, work on improving stress levels and maintaining proper eating habits during the luteal phase. Calcium, magnesium and bromelain, an enzyme found in pineapple, can help reduce cramping.

Feeling a heightened sense of intuition and clarity during this time? During menstruation, the left and right sides of the brain are both working well, so keep track of your thoughts and ideas at this time, perhaps keeping a journal close by so you can tap into your dreams or thoughts. As your symptoms start to improve and menstruation ends, don't be surprised if you feel anxious to get started on new plans and ideas.

The purpose of your four-phase cycle is to ovulate, aka make babies! As women, our bodies want to maintain a certain amount of fat and a perfect ratio of balanced hormones so that we can conceive with ease. But being fertile isn't just about making babies. If you have no interest in having children, you still want to maintain a healthy cycle and remain fertile for as long as possible; this is why suppressing your period with the birth control pill isn't always a good idea but is commonly the go-to for women who want to avoid pregnancy. The majority of the women I work with in my practice are either on the pill, have been on the pill or are thinking about coming off the pill. In some shape or form, the pill is always involved.

HERE'S WHAT YOU REALLY NEED TO KNOW ABOUT THE PILL

When you take birth control pills, you impose synthetic hormones on your natural cycle. Many birth control pills contain high levels of synthetic estrogen; it tricks your pituitary gland into thinking that you are pregnant and do not need to ovulate. Because your body thinks you are pregnant, the uterine lining thickens. Once you start the placebo pills in your pack, however, your estrogen level drops suddenly, and your body menstruates "normally." Or what you perceive to be normal.

The birth control pill suppresses ovulation. If you aren't ovulating, you are throwing off your entire hormonal system. Regular ovulation means you are fertile, your hormones are in check, and your cells and endocrine system are happy and functioning well. Plus, this is how your body produces estrogen and progesterone. The pill shuts down this entire process—the most important part of your 28-day cycle.

Most women think they are getting a regular period while they are on the pill, but that couldn't be further from the truth. The period that you experience while on the pill is referred to as a "pill-bleed." This abnormal cycle is what millions of women experience every month, and yet few doctors discuss the consequences of taking these prescriptions year after year.

THERE ARE REAL RISKS

Although I advise against hormonal contraceptives, if you choose to remain on the pill, I suggest you implement my post-pill supplement protocol to address any nutrient deficiencies. With that said, I do want to provide you with an overview of the reported risks and side effects of the birth control pill, because we are not often informed about these risks. Note that some physical and emotional changes take place that are permanent while you stay on the pill, and many of these changes occur as your body's response to synthetic estrogen. These changes include larger breasts, weight gain, reduced or increased acne, slight nausea, mood swings, irregular bleeding or spotting, breast tenderness and decreased libido.

Even scarier than the "mild" side effects are the serious health risks that accompany birth control pills, including:

- Increased risk of cervical and breast cancers
- Increased risk of heart attack and stroke
- Migraines
- Higher blood pressure
- Gallbladder disease
- Infertility
- Benign liver tumors
- Decreased bone density
- Yeast overgrowth and infection
- Increased risk of blood clotting
- Heart disease
- Polycystic ovary syndrome (PCOS)
- Insulin resistance

Birth control pills, as you can see, can truly wreak havoc on your health. And if that weren't enough, a scientific review published in 2016 found that progesterone-only contraceptives increased the incidence of skin conditions such as eczema, dermatitis and acne. Combined estrogen and progesterone contraceptives increased the risk of several autoimmune disorders such as multiple sclerosis (MS), ulcerative colitis, Crohn's disease and interstitial cystitis (painful bladder syndrome). This research was not limited to only oral contraceptives, but included both the NuvaRing and Mirena IUD.

One of the biggest areas the pill can affect is gut health. The pill can destroy beneficial bacteria in your intestines, making you more susceptible to yeast overgrowth, lowered immunity and infection. Let's take a deeper look at this, as well as the other areas it can impact.

1. **Digestion and Gut Health.** Taking synthetic hormones can impair the lining in your gut. A 2012 study linked birth control pills with a higher risk for inflammatory bowel diseases such as Crohn's and ulcerative colitis. Synthetic hormones change the permeability of the gut lining and synthetic estrogen does a number on the "good" bacteria in our gut. Keep in mind, your immune system "lives" in your gut. When the microbiome is impacted, your immune system will suffer as well.

2. **Inflammation.** Numerous studies show that women taking oral contraceptives have three times higher blood levels of C-reactive protein (CRP), a marker of chronic, systemic inflammation, than women who were not on the pill. High markers of inflammation are often associated with an increased risk in cancer, heart disease and diabetes. Whether you are on the pill or not, ask your doctor to test your high-sensitivity CRP (hs-CRP) so you can check your levels.

3. **Nutrient Deficiencies.** The pill messes with your gut's ability to adequately absorb B vitamins, specifically folate and vitamin B_{12}. It also inhibits the absorption of zinc and magnesium. These vitamins and minerals are crucial for liver support, detoxification and fertility.

If you want balanced, healthy hormones, your cycle is the first place to start. By following the nutrition, supplement and lifestyle protocols laid out in this book, you will be well on your way to optimized hormonal health. And if you're reading this while in your perimenopausal or postmenopausal years and you are no longer menstruating, the 30-Day Hormone Solution will help support your declining hormones and optimize your health in the best way possible.

I hope that you will feel more empowered to take charge of your health and hormones without the use of contraceptives—the very thing that crushes our libido, increases inflammation, depletes nutrients and blocks us from the very essence of our womanhood. There are other powerful and effective options for hormonal contraceptives. I suggest learning more about the fertility awareness method. For more information, check out *Taking Charge of Your Fertility* by Toni Weschler, the definitive guide to understanding natural contraception, and also look for *Beyond the Pill* by Dr. Jolene Brighten.

STOPPING HORMONAL BIRTH CONTROL

If you decide you want to come off hormonal birth control, there are some common symptoms you can expect, such as irregular or skipped periods, heavy menstrual bleeding, ovulation pain and menstrual cramps, acne, mood swings, bloating, water retention and nutrient deficiencies. Some women will get their periods back with no problem, but may still experience many of the other symptoms.

I know it can seem somewhat daunting to ditch the pill, especially if you are using it to help combat acne. I suffered with post-pill breakouts for a good six months, and I often hear from my clients that they'd rather go back on the pill than deal with acne. I get it, but please understand the harm you are doing to your body and how this will impact your future efforts to conceive. Keep in mind that if starting a family is a priority for you, what you do right now affects your fertility. The sooner you can come off the pill, the sooner you can start to reset your hormonal health and increase your chances of conceiving.

Here are the steps you need to take to reset your hormones post pill use. Keep in mind these supplements are great for daily use regardless of whether you've used hormonal contraceptives.

1. **Replenish Nutrient Deficiencies.** This includes supplementing with a good B-vitamin complex, vitamin C, vitamin D, zinc and magnesium. Ask your doctor to have your vitamin-D levels tested so you can see where you are within the range. Following the 30-Day Hormone Solution will support you in eating nutrient-rich foods in addition to daily supplementation. Adding in omega-3s is also important to help combat inflammation and support brain health, heart health and hormone production.

2. **Balance Your Blood Sugar.** We cover this extensively in Chapter 4 (page 44), and the 30-day meal plan is designed to help balance and support your blood sugar levels in the best way possible. Oral contraceptives have been linked with imbalanced blood sugar and insulin resistance, which is why many women experience post-pill PCOS. Balancing your meals with adequate amounts of protein, fat and non-starchy veggies, while eliminating white flour and wheat products, along with sugar, is the best way to support your blood sugar.

3. **Detox Estrogen and Support Your Gut.** Your liver metabolizes your hormones, so load up on liver-loving greens, such as dandelion, Swiss chard, kale, watercress, broccoli and other brassica vegetables as well as high-antioxidant foods, such as blueberries, raspberries and blackberries. You can also include liver-detox teas, such as dandelion or milk thistle. Restore gut health and optimize your microbiome by including a daily probiotic and eating fermented foods, such as sauerkraut, kimchi or coconut kefir. Fiber helps bind to toxins and excess estrogen in your body and flush it out, so eat ground flaxseeds and high-fiber fruits and vegetables.

4. **Use Targeted Herbs and Supplements.** Targeted herbs can vary based on your symptoms and condition. Vitex, also called chasteberry, helps regulate ovulation, increases fertility and improves progesterone. Vitamin C supports progesterone production and ovulation. Herbs such as rhodiola, holy basil and ashwagandha can improve cortisol production, lower inflammation and support the thyroid. Work with a practitioner to assess your specific needs and get on a targeted protocol.

The pill can have many serious unintended consequences. It can take time to restore your health and hormones post pill use and get back into a natural rhythm and flow with your cycle and hormones. Be patient with yourself and commit to a long-term plan. Resetting your hormonal health will take anywhere from three to twelve months post pill use. Implementing the strategies and protocols from this book will help you establish a new hormonal equilibrium and reclaim control over your body.

With that said, I feel it's important to discuss my foundational five supplements. I encourage you to include these throughout the 30-Day Hormone Solution for the best results. They will help to support your hormones, brain health, heart health, inflammation, gut health, energy, immune system, sleep and moods. These are the foundational five; add to this specific herbs or supplements that will further help to support your specific symptoms or issues (e.g., adrenal supplements, thyroid support, etc.).

FOUNDATIONAL FIVE SUPPLEMENTS	
Omega-3 Fish Oil	2 caps a day or 1 tablespoon (15 ml) of combined EPA and DHA of 1000+ mg
Probiotics	20–50 billion CFUs daily
Magnesium Bis-Glycinate	400 mg daily (before bed)
Vitamin D Liquid	5000 IU daily (or get tested to know your specific daily requirement)
Multivitamin OR PaleoGreens	2 capsules or 1 scoop daily

When it comes to vitamin D, it can be a challenge in North America to expose ourselves to sunlight daily—thanks to cold and long winters. I typically dose with a higher amount of vitamin D. It's important to get tested and then dose appropriately, making sure to retest after 2 to 3 months to adjust your dose. I have had only a handful of clients test within range for vitamin D, and most people are well below the range. Bottom line: Test—don't guess.

SEED CYCLING FOR BALANCED HORMONES

A simple and effective way to balance hormones using whole food nutrition is with seed cycling. Seed cycling is a way to help the body naturally balance its hormone levels by incorporating different seeds into the diet during the different phases of the menstrual cycle. By simply adding pumpkin seeds, flaxseeds, sunflower seeds or sesame seeds to your diet at the right time in your cycle, you can assist the body in either producing more of a needed hormone or processing and eliminating excess hormones.

FOLLICULAR PHASE (DAYS 1 TO 14)

Day 1 of your cycle is the day that menstruation begins. The two weeks that follow this make up the follicular phase. Pumpkin seeds and flaxseeds provide the body with omega-3 fatty acids, which promote healthy cell membranes, allowing hormones to reach their destinations within the body. Additionally, pumpkin seeds are high in zinc, which supports progesterone release, and flaxseeds contain lignans, which block excess estrogen. The combination of pumpkin and flaxseeds during phase 1 of your cycle helps balance estrogen production and absorption in the body.

During this phase, take 2 tablespoons (18 to 20 g) of raw pumpkin seeds and flaxseeds daily, in either oil or seed form. I recommended that you grind the seeds prior to consuming them to make sure that the lignans are adequately available for absorption

by your intestines. A coffee or herb grinder works great for this. You can add your oils or ground seeds to a smoothie or sip the oil right off the spoon.

LUTEAL PHASE (DAYS 15 TO 28)

Ovulation marks phase 2 of your cycle. It is typically around day 15—although not always. It marks a shift from estrogen production to progesterone production. During this phase, sesame seeds and sunflower seeds support the natural balance and production of hormones in the body. Sesame seeds, which also contain lignans, help block excess estrogen. Sunflower seeds provide the body with selenium, a trace mineral that assists the liver in detoxification and supports the thyroid.

During this phase, take 2 tablespoons (18 to 20 g) of raw sesame seeds and sunflower seeds daily, preferably ground. You can also include evening primrose oil as an omega-6 supplement, which is wonderful for easing PMS symptoms such as breast tenderness, menstrual cramps and mood swings.

The process of balancing your hormones naturally with seed cycling doesn't happen overnight. While you may begin to see changes sooner, it generally takes three months before you see significant changes in your symptoms. Be patient and take good care of yourself during this time by drinking lots of water, getting regular exercise and eating your greens!

How do you seed cycle if your period is irregular or missing? Simply by following the natural rhythm of the moon. The new moon would be day 1 of your period, while the full moon would be day 15. Pull out a moon calendar to see where in the month you are in the cycle and start tracking based on that.

If your cycle is missing or irregular or even if you have a regular cycle that is accompanied by PMS pain, I recommend seed cycling with a more therapeutic dose, as described on the next page.

THERAPEUTIC DOSES

- **New Moon to Full Moon:** 2,000 mg of flax oil three times daily with meals
- **Full Moon to New Moon:** 2,000 mg of primrose oil three times daily with meals

Once your menstrual cycle is fairly regulated, which could take anywhere from three months to a year, you can reduce your intake to a maintenance dose, as described below.

MAINTENANCE DOSES

- **New Moon to Full Moon:** 2,000 mg of flax oil once a day with breakfast
- **Full Moon to New Moon:** 2,000 mg of primrose oil once a day with breakfast

HORMONE-BALANCING SUPPLEMENTS

Dealing with hormonal imbalances can be complex. I recommend saliva hormone testing or the Dutch test to get to the bottom of complicated hormonal imbalances and provide you with a clearer picture of what is really going on with your hormones and symptoms. Then you can try some hormone-balancing supplements. Here are a few of my favorite brands that I recommend:

FOR ESTROGEN DOMINANCE

- DIM-Evail by Design for Health
- Calcium D-Glucarate by Design for Health or XYMOGEN
- Probiotics by Design for Health, Mega-SporeBiotic, Renew Life or Genuine Health
- BroccoProtect by Design for Health

FOR PAINFUL PERIODS

- Turmeric by Integrative Therapeutics
- Omega-3 fish oil by NutraSea or Design for Health
- Magnesium Bis-Glycinate by CanPrev or Design for Health
- Crampbark by St. Francis Herb Farm

FOR SHORT CYCLES (UNDER 24 DAYS)

- Fémance Chastetree by St. Francis Herb Farm
- Adrenotone by Design for Health

FOR PMS

- Adrenotone by Design for Health
- Magnesium Bis-Glycinate by CanPrev or Design for Health
- Omega-3 fish oil by NutraSea or Design for Health
- Vitamin D liquid by Design for Health, Can-Prev or Advanced Orthomolecular Research
- B-Supreme by Design for Health
- Hormone complex blends: ESTROsmart, EstroSense or Harmony Balance

FOR MENOPAUSE

- Turmeric by Integrative Therapeutics
- Omega-3 fish oil by NutraSea or Design for Health
- Magnesium Bis-Glycinate by CanPrev or Design for Health
- Hormone complex blends: Harmony Menopause, Harmony Menopause Max or MenoSense

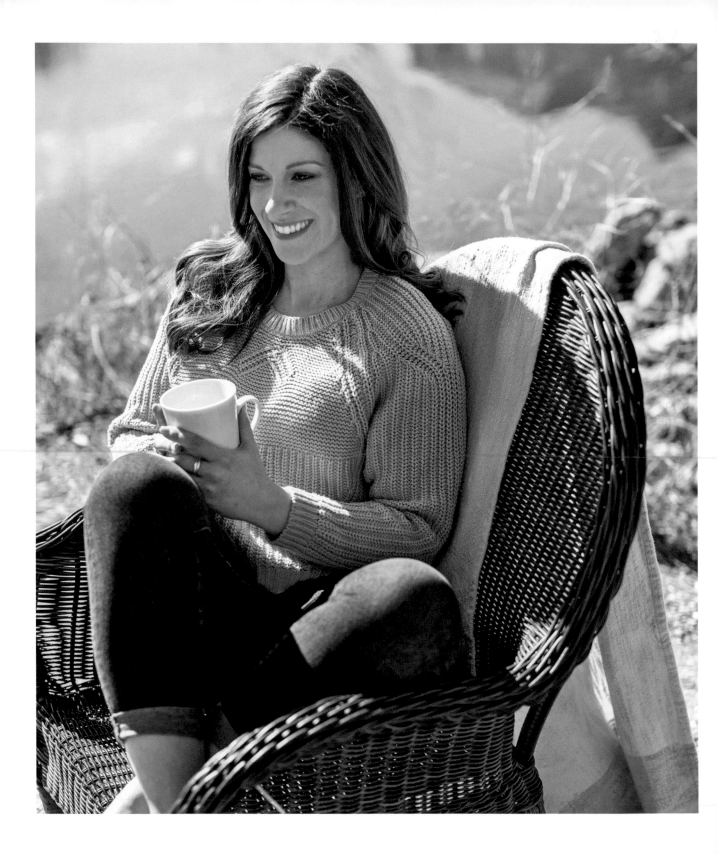

CHAPTER 3:

CORTISOL AND YOUR THYROID:

FEELING FAT, FATIGUED AND INFLAMED?

Have you heard of the adrenal glands? They are two little glands that sit on top of your kidneys. And, although they are tiny, they sure are mighty. Your adrenals control quite a few actions in your body, including your stress response, weight, blood sugar, blood pressure and immune system. In fact, they are our primary survival organs. But they can also be responsible for feeling unwell—from weight gain to irritability, fatigue, blood sugar irregularities and low thyroid function, your adrenals can cause you to experience multiple symptoms, which we commonly refer to as adrenal fatigue.

YOUR ADRENAL GLANDS

Adrenal fatigue is a term that we use quite frequently and rather loosely in the health and wellness field. More accurately speaking, what we're referring to is dysfunction of the hypothalamic-pituitary-adrenal (HPA) axis. Your adrenals communicate with your brain and vice versa. When you are exposed to certain triggers, such as blood sugar highs or lows, environmental toxins, perceived stress, poor-quality sleep, blue light pollution, circadian rhythm disruption and gut inflammation, you impair the communication between the brain and the adrenals. In turn, your adrenals aren't getting sent the right hormones they need, and what you feel is adrenal fatigue, or rather, symptoms such as:

- Exhaustion
- Low thyroid function
- Weight gain
- Sleep disturbances
- Lack of focus and concentration
- Sugar cravings

Hormonal balance is essential to good health, and the adrenal glands are center stage in the body's ability to regulate hormones. In fact, roughly 70 to 80 percent of all doctor visits are for stress-related conditions for which doctors have little or no training and nothing to offer other than temporary relief care.

Our adrenal glands control our fight-or-flight response. When we are in danger, or when there is a perceived danger or threat, our adrenals kick into high gear and mobilize all our resources so we can fight or flee from danger.

Historically speaking, our immediate dangers were rather short-lived—think running from a tiger or lion in the jungle. Nowadays, in our concrete jungle, we are dealing with daily stressors of bills and finances, relationships, work, bosses, careers, piles of projects, a heavy workload and being stuck in traffic. Not to mention an overconsumption of caffeine to get us going! Our perceived daily stressors are nothing in comparison to outrunning a tiger in the jungle, yet we are constantly reacting—or overreacting—and worrying about 80 percent of things that don't even happen! Our need for cortisol and adrenaline is at an all-time high.

When our HPA axis gets activated, we pump out a hormone called cortisol—a no-nonsense, strategic-thinking hormone. It alerts our nervous system to threats, helps regulate our hormones and gets much-needed blood sugar to our muscles so we can fight or flee. I'm sure we've all experienced the high of cortisol before—heavy breathing, sweating, increased heart rate and high energy. Insulin is another hormone involved in this process. It comes along to mop up the excess mobilized blood sugar back into your cells, allowing your heart rate and breathing to get back to normal. And then—all is well, and we go on our merry way.

In nature, constant stress is rare, but in our human world, we are dealing with all kinds of stressors, pushing our adrenals into overdrive and impairing the communication between the adrenals and the brain. This is what leads to burnout and exhaustion. The problem is, other hormones are impacted as well. Not only are you forcing your body to pump out excess cortisol, but excess blood sugar and insulin, which, over time, can lead to insulin resistance and weight gain. Ever wondered where all those cravings for fat, sugar and salt came from? Yup—from your daily stressors!

Cortisol gets a bad rap, when it really helps us bounce back from our daily stressors. Without cortisol we would die. It's just that we don't want too little or too much of it. We want it in the right amount. Over time, unrelenting stress can cause us to burn out our adrenals, where we go from overproducing cortisol, to underproducing it.

So, what are some signs and symptoms that your adrenals are burnt out?

1. You have difficulty falling asleep, staying asleep and do not feel rested upon waking.

2. You're craving fat, sugar and salt.

3. Your memory and focus are lacking.

4. You're experiencing digestive issues.

5. You feel irritable and anxious.

6. You get tired most afternoons around 3 to 4 p.m. and crave sugar, salt or are looking for a caffeine fix.

7. You're gaining weight—primarily around your waist.

8. Your hormones are a mess—from PMS to infertility and low libido.

9. You get sick more often and have a hard time recovering.

10. You anger quickly and find yourself snappy.

11. You have low thyroid function.

There are different stages of adrenal fatigue, and you can always test your adrenals with a salivary or urine test for a better understanding of how they are functioning. The best testing looks at a 24-hour range so you can see where your peaks and dips of cortisol occur through the day, which can provide you with clues as to what might be going on to trigger these fluctuations.

- **Stage 1—Wired and Tired:** In this stage, your cortisol levels are naturally elevated in the morning. However, you feel wired and tired, which is characterized by elevated cortisol at night when it should be low. This leads to difficulty falling asleep and often, people in this stage may also regularly feel "on edge."

- **Stage 2—Stressed and Tired:** The second stage shows more severe cortisol disruption with higher cortisol in the morning but falling quickly after lunch, leading to afternoon fog and tiredness. You may get a second wind at night, but most often wake in the middle of the night and are unable to fall back asleep.

- **Stage 3—Full Burnout:** If you've ever had a baby (I have not), the symptoms in this stage can be compared to how a woman feels in early pregnancy or with a newborn—exhausted all the time! Your cortisol patterns are completely disrupted, putting you at higher risk of thyroid disease, autoimmune disease and gut problems.

ADRENALS AND YOUR THYROID

Stress and your adrenals are intricately connected to your thyroid health. I can surely attest to this! If you are in a stressed state, the adrenals will be "up" and the thyroid will be "down"—you can't have both going at the same time. In other words, if you have a low-functioning thyroid, it means you have high-functioning adrenals. There are many ways to support both your adrenals and thyroid. In fact, when supporting your thyroid, it's essential to also support your adrenals. I'm often asked, Which one do I treat first? Often, it's both!

When your body is in fight-or-flight mode, your normal functions are deprioritized. Anything that is not necessary for overcoming your perceived stressor does not need to function. This means your digestion, your immune response and your thyroid. Your thyroid function is temporarily put on hold or slowed down until your stress has passed. Ideally, we hope that this is an acute stress and not chronic, so that your body can return to optimal function as quickly as possible.

Unfortunately, today we are dealing with daily chronic stressors. Perhaps we have an ongoing stressor, or one stressor followed by another. This ongoing demand for cortisol has a negative impact on your thyroid. Because your adrenals speak with your hypothalamus and pituitary gland in your brain, these glands also regulate your thyroid hormone. If they are busy dealing with the adrenals, they can't also regulate thyroid hormone production. These glands, when under chronic stress, work to conserve your thyroid hormone output.

Not only that, but stress hormones can put the brakes on your thyroid output, leading to symptoms of hypothyroid (aka low thyroid function). It's important to note that your immune system will also be suppressed when your body is in stress mode, which can trigger latent viral infections, some of which can trigger autoimmune thyroid disease. The suppressing of your immune system means that your primary immune barriers, such as the blood-brain barrier, lungs and gut barrier, are also weakened. I'm sure you've heard the term "leaky gut," which can be a trigger for autoimmune disease and releases pathogens, toxins, gluten and dairy, among other things, into your bloodstream.

HEALING YOUR ADRENALS

It's important to take active steps to heal your adrenals. The following are some time-tested ways to calm your nervous system.

RELAXATION

Including relaxation techniques, such as meditation or mindfulness, can activate your parasympathetic nervous system (relaxed state) and deactivate your sympathetic nervous system (fight-or-flight response). This will help your body to pump out *fewer* stress hormones and can truly help your adrenals heal and restore themselves.

REAL TALK

When it comes to healing your adrenal glands there is no quick fix. You can't just pop a pill and call it a day. Healing your adrenals takes time and includes taking radical responsibility for how you show up in your life and for yourself. It's the lifestyle shifts that have the biggest impact on your adrenal health. The best treatment doesn't include fancy herbs or supplements or some magical superfood; it is simply practicing relaxation.

I know, it's easier said than done. I can't tell you how many times I've sat down to meditate and 30 seconds in, my monkey brain is going and I'm thinking about what to order off of Amazon! You have to find the meditation that works for you. Consider looking into yoga nidra, or download a meditation app such as Headspace. The HeartMath Inner Balance app is another great option, as it uses an external sensor on your earlobe to help you synchronize your heart rate, breath and mind. There are so many options out there, so start looking for some apps or tools that will work for you.

INFRARED SAUNA THERAPY

Spending time in an infrared sauna—which I address in more detail in Chapter 7, page 77—has many health benefits, including stress relief and detoxification. Plus, it's a great time to sit in peace and quiet for twenty minutes with some soothing music or your meditation app. Consider purchasing one for your home or finding a local spa in your area that has one.

RELAXING HOT BATH

I love winding down at the end of the day with a hot bath. I add some Epsom salts and lavender oil, and dim the lights or light some candles. It's a great way to activate your parasympathetic nervous system, plus it's also wonderful for detoxification. A hot bath can also help improve your sleep, which is often lacking when there is chronic stress going on.

SLEEP

Speaking of sleep, it is essential to healing your adrenals and overall hormonal health. When I first started on my autoimmune healing protocol, which contains many of the strategies discussed in this book, I was sleeping for nine or ten hours a night for the first few weeks. My body needed it. Practice sleep hygiene and create healthy boundaries around your sleep; going to bed at the same time every night and waking at the same time can do wonders for your stress.

DITCH THE SUGAR AND CAFFEINE

There is no shortage of energy bars, organic coffees, green teas, energy elixirs and shots and sugar bombs. The problem is, these do not fix our energy problems for very long. I'm all for a cup of coffee, but if you are burnt out and can't sleep, then your cup of joe has got to go—at least temporarily while you work on healing your adrenals and hormones. I cut coffee out completely while working on healing my thyroid, and then I slowly introduced decaf and then full caffeine. I also pay attention to my stress level and workload, being conscious not to overconsume coffee while dealing with acute or chronic stressors. Sugar and coffee—I should also add wine to the mix!—will put you on a roller coaster of sugar highs and lows, ultimately leading to energy depletion. Give them the boot, work on healing and then slowly reintroduce them.

HERBS AND SUPPLEMENTS

On top of creating lifestyle shifts, adaptogenic herbs can be a wonderful addition to an adrenal healing protocol. They help the body adapt and cope with stress and work to support, nourish and replenish the adrenals, whether they are on overdrive or fatigued. Some of my favorite herbs and supplements for women include the following:

Ashwagandha is calming, helps with muscle aches, promotes sleep and helps with T4 to T3 conversion.

- **Dose:** 3 to 6 grams of the dried herb in capsule form daily OR 1 to 4 ml (20 to 80 drops) of tincture, in water, 3 times daily
- **Cautions:** Not for use during pregnancy. Use cautiously if you are sensitive to plants in the nightshade family. Avoid with pharmaceutical sedatives and pain medications.

Rhodiola is also wonderful, especially if you have anxiety or issues with mental focus.

- **Dose:** 200 to 400 mg in capsules or tablets daily OR 2 to 3 ml (40 to 60 drops) of tincture, in water, 2 to 3 times daily. Use products standardized to 2 to 3 percent rosavin and 0.8 to 1 percent salidroside.
- **Cautions:** Avoid if you have bipolar depression with manic behavior.

Holy basil is great, especially for those who need extra immune support. I personally love drinking holy basil tea at night before bed.

- **Dose:** 2 to 3 ml (40 to 60 drops) of tincture, in water, 3 times daily
- **Cautions:** None known

Shatavari is also an incredible adaptogen. In Ayurvedic medicine it is known as the "queen of herbs." It is both nourishing and calming and great for hormonal balancing, specifically if you have PMS, mood swings or menopausal symptoms. I find it also works great as a fertility tonic and is helpful for those dealing with low libido.

- **Dose:** 2 to 4 ml (40 to 80 drops) of tincture, in water, 2 to 3 times daily
- **Cautions:** Avoid if you have a history of estrogen-receptor positive cancer.

Reishi mushrooms deserve an honorable mention. I absolutely love medicinal mushrooms for their powerful immune support, anticancer properties and antifungal benefits. Reishi, in particular, is great for nourishing and supporting the adrenal glands. It's also wonderful for modulating the immune system and helping your body better handle or resist the common cold or flu. It also works to reduce inflammation in the body. Overall, reishi is great for calming the nervous system, promoting deeper sleep and supporting the body's natural abilities to detoxify.

- **Dose:** 3 to 9 grams of the dried mushroom in capsules or tablets daily OR 2 to 4 ml of reishi tincture, in water 2 to 3 times daily
- **Cautions:** Avoid with blood thinners and medications that lower blood pressure, based on theoretical risks of drug interactions.

B vitamins are critical for the chemical processes within the adrenal glands and are involved in every neurological process in the body. A B-complex supplement would be great for the adrenals.

Omega-3 fatty acids, vitamin C and **magnesium** are also beneficial for the adrenals.

Some of my favorite brands that contain the herbs on the previous page in a complex form are Designs for Health Adrenotone, Gaia Herbs Adrenal Health, Advanced Orthomolecular Research Ortho-Adapt, St. Francis Herb Farm Stress tincture or PURICA Complete 360, which is a blend of multiple medicinal mushrooms plus adaptogenic herbs. PURICA Immune 7 is also a wonderful product that contains a blend of seven medicinal mushrooms.

THE IMPORTANCE OF YOUR THYROID

What if I were to tell you that just about every conventional doctor overlooks—or should I say, ignores—one incredibly common health problem that affects 200 million people worldwide and can be the cause of any symptom under the sun? That, my friend, is your thyroid.

HOW THE THYROID FUNCTIONS

The thyroid, a butterfly-shaped gland in the center of your neck, is the master gland of your metabolism. How well your thyroid is functioning is interrelated with every system in your body: your brain, your lungs, digestion and your ovaries. If your thyroid is not running optimally, then neither are you—and you will feel its effects. Let's take a quick look at how the thyroid functions.

Thyroid stimulating hormone (TSH) is produced by your pituitary gland in your brain. Its job is to tell the thyroid gland that it's time to produce more thyroid hormone. Once your thyroid gland receives this message and it's functioning well and healthy, it produces two hormones—triiodothyronine (T3) and thyroxine (T4).

T4 is your inactive thyroid hormone. It floats around your bloodstream and truthfully, doesn't do too much on its own. What your body really needs is T3, the active thyroid hormone. Your liver pulls on some of the reserve T4 and converts it into T3. As your cells use up your T3, your body detects this decrease in circulating T3 and draws even more from your T4 reserves. Your brain, specifically your hypothalamus, notices that T3 and T4 supplies are dwindling and it starts this process all over again. If your body wants to conserve energy, rather than burn it, it will divert your active T3 to its inactive form, rT3, which is its "reserve" form. A high level of rT3 is usually a signal of an underactive thyroid (hypothyroidism). On the flip side, too much thyroid hormone will lead to an overactive thyroid (hyperthyroidism), which throws your metabolism into high gear.

Like all of our hormones, having them present in the right amounts will ensure we feel great and experience incredible health. But optimizing your thyroid function can often be a challenge because it's innately connected to so many other glands in your body—the hypothalamus, the pituitary and the adrenals. There is a chain of command or communication that is intelligently happening in your body in order for your thyroid to function, and it starts with your hypothalamus giving the green light to your pituitary.

Problems can arise at any point during this communication. Often there can be a problem converting T4 into T3 as a result of emotional or physiological stress, restricting food intake, excessive exercise, overeating, inflammation or nutrient deficiencies.

SYMPTOMS OF LOW THYROID FUNCTION

Are you experiencing constipation, weight gain, headaches, fatigue, mood swings, irritability, PMS, irregular cycles and sleep disturbances? There's a good chance it's your thyroid. In fact, the number of women who visit their doctor yearly with these exact complaints only to be handed an antidepressant and some birth control is alarming!

Hypothyroidism, or low thyroid function, is a common condition in North America that affects between roughly 20 to 25 percent of the female population. Only about 10 percent of the male population tends to be affected. In fact, more than 30 percent of women over the age of 35 have subclinical or mild hypothyroidism, where their TSH (thyroid stimulating hormone) is within normal range, yet they still experience symptoms of low thyroid function. Common symptoms of hypothyroidism include:

- Constipation
- Headaches
- Weight gain
- Depression and irritability
- Hair loss
- Heart palpitations
- Brain fog and memory loss
- Poor vision
- Fatigue and weakness
- Cold hands and feet
- Hormonal imbalances such as PMS, irregular cycle or infertility, fibroids, menopausal symptoms and miscarriage
- Insomnia

SYMPTOMS OF HIGH THYROID FUNCTION

Although hypothyroidism is more common, we do not want to overlook hyperthyroid, which can usually be a result of Graves' disease, an autoimmune condition. Common symptoms of hyperthyroidism include:

- Rapid heart rate
- Sweating
- Weight loss
- Irritability
- Shakiness
- Insomnia
- Anxiety
- Issues with bone density and loss of muscle mass

GETTING TO THE BOTTOM OF THYROID TESTING

Statistically speaking, hypothyroidism is an underdiagnosed condition due to outdated lab testing. Unfortunately, most doctors only test TSH and consider your thyroid function to be normal if your test range falls between 0.4 and 5.0 IU/ml. This reference range may vary based on different countries. In functional and naturopathic medicine, the new norm for TSH lab value is between 0.4 and 2.0 IU/ml. TSH is a moving target and can often be misleading, as levels of circulating hormones may fluctuate at different times.

This makes me think of my client Elise, a 41-year-old woman with heavier than normal periods, extreme fatigue, constipation, sleep disturbances and constant waking through the night. She had a 10-pound (4.5-kg) weight gain in a matter of two months. These are all signs of low thyroid function. She asked her primary care doctor to check her thyroid labs, and lo and behold, her TSH (which was all that was tested) came back within the normal range (4.2 UL/ml)—although at the high end. She was told her thyroid was fine and sent on her way.

The truth is her labs weren't normal. This is hypothyroidism, and it warrants further testing and investigation. In fact, 95 percent of hypothyroidism is due to autoimmune Hashimoto's, and it is important to rule out Hashimoto's by testing your thyroid antibodies.

AUTOIMMUNE HASHIMOTO'S

While the name sounds a lot like a sushi dish, Hashimoto's is an autoimmune condition. It is the leading cause of hypothyroidism, and it is silently destroying lives. Back in 2017, I started to notice some interesting symptoms. My hands had these strange aching pains and stiffness. My fatigue was taking over, and I felt like a walking zombie. My brain was foggy, and my memory was failing me. And then my sleep started to suffer.

You might be thinking, "But Samantha, you're a nutritionist and you eat so well. How could this be?!" Yes, I eat well and exercise and practice what I preach, but I am also a human being who is running a business, has a crazy to-do list, deals with personal and professional stressors and has a constant monkey in my brain. You see, stress is stress. Your body can't differentiate between a tragic stress, such as a death in the family, from a common stress, such as a to-do list with 25 things on it. A busy brain is a stressed brain, and I've definitely had my fair share of overwhelm when it comes to running a business. It's safe to say that my stress exacerbated my symptoms, causing my immune system to go haywire.

In addition, there is a history of autoimmunity in my family. My mother has an autoimmune condition, as did my grandmother and so do all of my female cousins on my mother's side of the family. There is definitely a genetic disposition linked to my Hashimoto's.

Plus, I had issues with my gut health. My digestion and gut have always been an area of weakness for me. I was a C-section baby and I was formula fed. Being a C-section baby means you don't pass through the birth canal to pick up all that good beneficial bacteria and, of course, not being breast-fed meant I didn't get the essential nutrients and goodness that only breast milk provides.

I was also put on numerous over-the-counter meds and pharmaceuticals as a kid. Whether it was a cough or sniffle, my parents were quick to open the Benadryl. My parents did what they knew best, and they were completely unaware about naturopathic and natural medicine. But it's important to note how these things—which may seem minor—can have such a huge impact on your immune system, gut health and genetic expression.

6 THYROID LABS TO LOOK AT

TEST NAME	STANDARD REFERENCE RANGE	OPTIMAL REFERENCE RANGE
TSH	0.4 TO 5.0 IU/ML	0.4 TO 2.0 IU/ML
FREE T4	9 TO 23 PMOL/L	15 TO 23 PMOL/L
FREE T3	3 TO 7 PMOL/L	5 TO 7 PMOL/L
REVERSE T3	11 TO 21 NG/DL	11 TO 18 NG/DL
TPO ANTIBODIES	< 35 IU/ML	< 2 IU/ML
TG ANTIBODIES	< 35 IU/ML	< 2 IU/ML

In fact, Dr. Alessio Fasano, a world-renowned gastroenterologist, discovered that there are three factors that cause an autoimmune disease to manifest:

- Genetic predisposition
- An environmental trigger, such as stress or a toxin (i.e., heavy metals)
- Intestinal permeability (i.e., leaky gut)

Check, check and check.

Hashimoto's is more an autoimmune condition than it is a thyroid condition—like I said, it *triggers* hypothyroidism. An autoimmune disease occurs when your immune system attacks healthy cells. This can occur anywhere in your body, from your thyroid to your joints, kidneys or gastrointestinal tract. This can often lead to multiple autoimmune conditions at one given time, where your immune system goes on to attack more than one area. Autoimmunity can be challenging to diagnose, given that there are more than 80 different types, many of which have very similar symptoms.

Many of the women I coach in my private practice are quick to dive in and work on only their thyroid, but you have to keep in mind that autoimmune Hashimoto's is not just a thyroid issue. It's an immune issue, and that is why gut health and environmental triggers need to be addressed. There is a lot you can do to get your autoimmune condition into remission using nutrition, supplementation and lifestyle factors.

By following the strategies laid out in this book you'll be optimizing the health of your thyroid. If you do have Hashimoto's, consider looking into the AIP diet (Autoimmune Paleo Protocol), a powerful strategy that uses diet and lifestyle to regulate the immune system, putting an end to these attacks and giving the body the opportunity to heal. The AIP diet cuts out all the potential triggering foods that would aggravate your gut and immune system.

AIP can come with many restrictions; it is often seen as the "stricter" version of the Paleo diet. But it truly is worth following if you are suffering with an autoimmune condition. I followed it for a good six weeks with tremendous results. With that said, start here with my 30-Day Hormone Solution, eliminate grains, gluten, dairy, sugar, beans and legumes. Then move into the AIP diet for further elimination. If you're looking for more information about the AIP protocol, head on over to www.holisticwellness.ca/aipprotocol for more information.

When it comes to healing your autoimmune Hashimoto's, there are eight key strategies to have in place. Note that these strategies are essential for all your hormones. The good news is that we cover it all in this book! Proper testing is at the top of this list, as it is essential to know your thyroid numbers and have them interpreted by a practitioner who can help you understand them. Many conventional doctors do not test for Hashimoto's antibodies. If you want to rule out whether or not you have Hashimoto's, it's essential to have your antibodies tested. The higher your antibody levels, the higher the attack on your thyroid.

1. Get the proper testing.
2. Eat protein + fat + fiber (PFF) meals.
3. Avoid gluten.
4. Eat carbs—the right kinds.
5. Monitor your exercise.
6. Use appropriate supplementation.
7. Heal your gut.
8. Manage stress.

THYROID SUPPLEMENTS

There are many supplements that can be beneficial for supporting the thyroid gland. It's important to always work on healing the root cause of your thyroid disease. Let's take a look at some thyroid supplement essentials.

Vitamin D$_3$ functions more like a hormone in your body, and it is an important immune modulator. Studies show that those with hypothyroidism tend to have significantly lower levels of vitamin D. I suggest having your vitamin D$_3$ levels tested so you can better gauge what dose to supplement with.

- **Typical Dose:** 2,000–5,000 IU/day, depending on your serum levels. Ideally, recheck your blood levels eight weeks after starting supplementation to determine whether you are on your optimal dose. Vitamin D$_3$ is safe during pregnancy and breastfeeding, and it should be included as part of a pre-pregnancy plan and protocol.
- **Cautions:** None known

Selenium is critical for thyroid health. It assists with the conversion of T4 to T3, and it has been shown to decrease the risk of developing postpartum thyroiditis in women who are positive for TPO antibodies before or during pregnancy. Your body works to turn selenium into glutathione, the powerful antioxidant that protects your thyroid from inflammation and oxidative stress. Food sources include Brazil nuts, lamb, turkey, eggs, cod and mushrooms.

- **Typical Dose:** 200 mcg/day. Do not exceed that amount unless working with a practitioner.
- **Cautions:** Selenium can worsen thyroid function if you're also experiencing iodine deficiency. Make sure you know your iodine status before starting selenium.

Zinc is an important mineral that is involved in the conversion of T4 to T3. In one study, participants who took zinc sulfate for twelve months had T3 levels come into the normal range. They also had decreases in reverse T3, and they had better communication between the hypothalamus and the thyroid. Zinc is also important for both male and female fertility. I typically recommend taking it with copper. Try the Zinc-Copper Balance by Advanced Orthomolecular Research.

- **Typical Dose:** 30 mg/day. Take with meals to prevent nausea. Zinc is safe when pregnant and breastfeeding.
- **Cautions:** None known

Ashwagandha is not only great for adrenal health, but research also shows that it helps increase circulating T4 levels with no influence on T3. Research also suggests that ashwagandha may benefit the liver; and because that's where T4 to T3 conversion largely happens, perhaps this explains some of the benefits of ashwagandha.

- **Typical Dose:** 3 to 6 grams of the dried herb in capsule form daily OR 1 to 4 ml (20 to 80 drops) of tincture, in water, 3 times daily
- **Cautions:** Do not use during pregnancy. Use cautiously if you are sensitive to plants in the nightshade family. Avoid with pharmaceutical sedatives and pain medications.

Inositol. Recent research has discovered that the combination of selenium (200 mcg/day) and inositol—specifically myoinositol—is even more powerful at reducing both anti-TPO and anti-Tg antibodies. The combination also does more to improve thyroid function and TSH levels than selenium alone. Six months of treatment was needed in order to see improvement, and participants even reported better quality of life overall.

- **Typical Dose:** 600 mg/day, which is safe during pregnancy and breastfeeding. I recommend staying on this combination at least until thyroid antibodies are normalized, which could take roughly 6 to 8 months, or remain on it indefinitely if needed.
- **Cautions:** None known

THYROID MEDICATION

While medication can be necessary in some cases, women are being prescribed thyroid medications even when their T4 and T3 are completely fine. In addition, most conventional medical doctors are prescribing medications such as Synthroid or levothyroxine without running a full thyroid panel, and then getting their patients on these medications for years and years without any follow-up!

I've seen it happen too many times while working with my clients. For example, take Ann, a 46-year-old woman who came to see me specifically looking to lose 30 pounds (13.6 kg). She was also experiencing fatigue, brain fog, sleeplessness and joint pain. She had been on Synthroid for nearly twenty years, without any change to her dose or follow-up regarding her thyroid. I sent her to have her full thyroid panel tested and sure enough, her antibodies were extremely high, confirming that she had Hashimoto's. Working with her and another naturopath, we switched her over to natural desiccated thyroid and put her on the 30-Day Hormone Solution. She lost 12 pounds (5.4 kg) within the first three weeks. Ann has gone on to lose more weight, and her brain fog and joint pain have subsided. She continues to follow an anti-inflammatory diet, monitors her thyroid antibodies and gets regular thyroid panels tested every four to six months.

There are different brands of desiccated thyroid, and they also vary based on whether you live in Canada or the United States. Speak with your naturopath or functional medical doctor about the best approach, dose and brand for you. Natural desiccated thyroid contains both T4 and T3, while most generic medications, such as Synthroid or levothyroxine, contain only T4. Remember, T3 is your active thyroid hormone, which is why most women tend to feel better on a combination of T4 and T3. There are also T3-only options available. Ask your doctor or practitioner about Nature-Throid, WP Thyroid, NDT (also known as ERFA in Canada) or Armour. And keep in mind, some people do better on Synthroid or levothyroxine, and there's nothing wrong with that. What's important is that you know you have options and to seek out other treatments that will serve you and your health best.

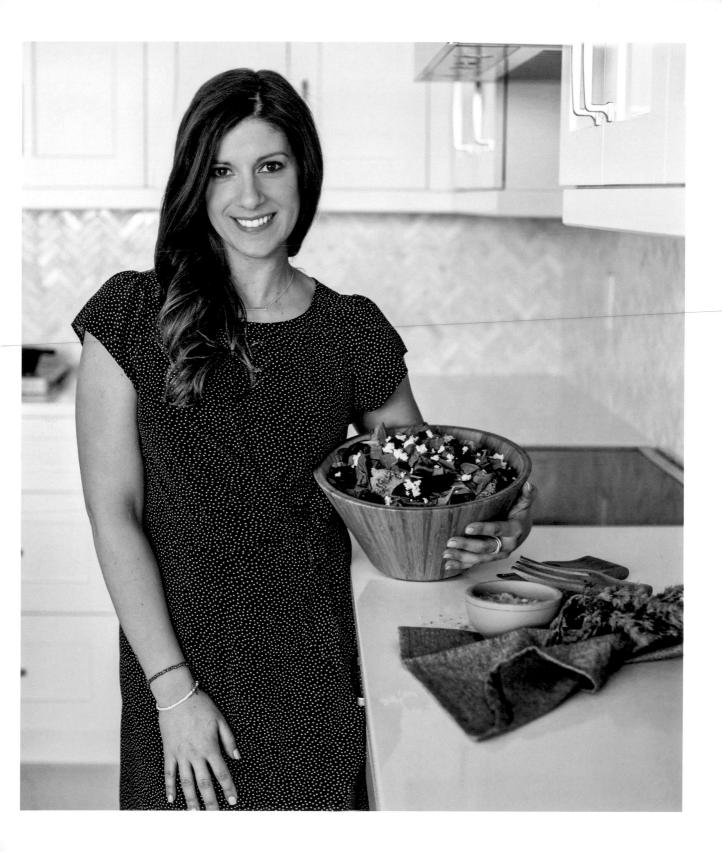

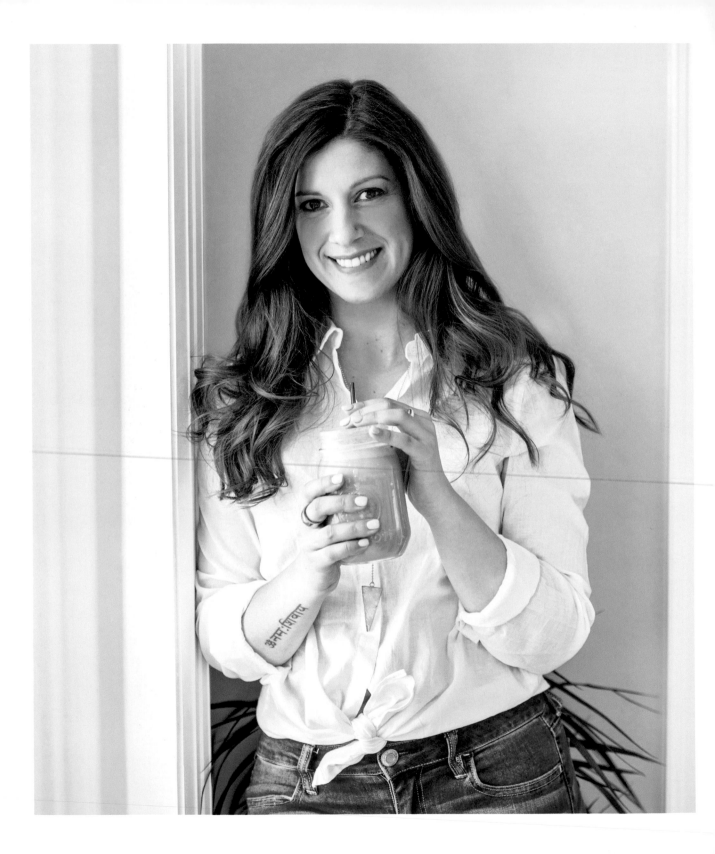

CHAPTER 4:

INSULIN AND BLOOD SUGAR:

THE MASTER TO HORMONAL HARMONY

Have you ever felt irritable, anxious or moody for no reason? As though out of nowhere you suddenly stepped into this alter ego that was mean as heck?

You can thank your blood sugar for that. In fact, I'm sure you've heard the term "hangry" before. It means being both hungry and angry at the same time. It's not a pretty sight. The good news is that it can be fixed once you've eaten something. Your energy comes back. Your alter ego subsides, and she even feels bad for being snappy at the women in the checkout line a few minutes ago.

But then she returns. It's two hours after you've eaten lunch and your hangry alter ego is back with a vengeance. Looking for something sweet. Maybe a coffee? A muffin? But you ate not too long ago, so why is she back?

If you sat down to lunch and filled yourself up with a bowl of rice, some teriyaki chicken covered in some creamy sauce and a splattering of chopped veggies, then there's good reason why your alter ego has returned. You're missing adequate protein and fat, two macronutrients that keep your blood sugar stable, your mood balanced and your mind sharp. You're also missing a healthy dose of fiber that keeps you satiated for longer.

And so, you reach for that muffin or coffee, or maybe both. You head back to your desk, and you find yourself hangry again two hours later.

Perhaps your hangry ride on the blood sugar roller coaster has taught you to eat every two to three hours to stay balanced. And when you don't eat every two to three hours you feel it—irritable, anxious and moody. Plus, isn't eating every few hours the sweet spot for weight loss? Eating small frequent meals all day long means we are stoking our metabolism, right?

Unfortunately, this couldn't be further from the truth. Let's take a deep dive into insulin and blood sugar to understand why eating more frequently is actually hindering your weight loss efforts.

IS SNACKING MAKING YOU FAT?

Your pancreas produces insulin. Insulin is the hardworking hormone that seeks out sugar, also known as glucose, and turns it into useful energy. When you eat a meal, sugar enters your bloodstream in the form of glucose. Your pancreas secretes insulin to manage the sugar in your blood and transport the sugar to your cells. Once at your cells, insulin basically knocks on the cell door and asks to enter with sugar in tow.

In a healthy body, the cell doors will hear the knock and open the door. On the other hand, if you are consuming a high-carbohydrate diet and not exercising, this process doesn't always happen and the cell door won't answer the knock. If you are constantly forcing insulin to overwork and knock on the cell doors, your pancreas and your fat cells become exhausted over time.

Your pancreas is one tough little bugger, and when your cells won't open their door to insulin, your pancreas is forced to produce *even more* insulin in an effort to get the sugar through the cell door.

When your cells no longer respond to insulin, this is what is called insulin resistance. It's the precursor to diabetes. Basically, your cells have lost their ability to detect and store glucose, making them resistant. In fact, it's one of the leading causes of polycystic ovary syndrome (PCOS) and one of the main reasons why women experience terrible PMS, mood swings, headaches and weight gain. High insulin levels can stimulate the ovaries to overproduce testosterone. This is why women with PCOS tend to suffer with cystic acne and facial hair growth. By managing insulin, you can manage the overproduction of testosterone.

Insulin resistance can be caused by poor gut and liver health, depleted gut flora (good bacteria), and by inflammation caused by the overconsumption of inflammatory foods such as sugar, a high-carb diet and processed vegetable oils.

If you are eating every two to three hours, not only are you forcing your pancreas to produce more insulin throughout the day, but you're also constantly knocking on your cell doors, hoping to let sugar into your cells. Can you see how this would pose a problem? Over time, as your cells become insulin resistant, insulin has to go somewhere. And so, it builds up in the bloodstream, and this causes a host of issues and increases inflammation, also leading to low libido and infertility.

To balance your blood sugar and insulin levels, eating every two to three hours is *not the answer.* You should be able to go at least four to six hours between meals *without* feeling jittery, moody and hangry.

Chronically high levels of insulin also make it extremely difficult, if not impossible, to lose weight. When you're eating every two to three hours, what your body is actually doing is burning through glycogen (stored sugar). To burn adipose tissue (fat), you need to stretch out that time frame closer to five hours, *the sweet spot.*

Really, when you think about it, were we ever designed to eat five or six meals a day, every two to three hours? If we think back to the Paleolithic era, there wasn't an abundance of food. We followed a feast-or-famine type of "diet."

Breakfast, lunch and dinner were the norm. Not breakfast, snack, lunch, snack, dinner, snack. I mean, who has time to prep all that food anyway?! Three meals a day is effective for weight loss and balancing hormones, and it's exactly the plan you'll be following for your 30-day program. How many times on a Saturday have you slept in, had a large brunch, went about your day running errands and then, before you knew it, it was 6 p.m. and time for dinner? You've probably had many laid-back weekends where you ate only two meals a day.

Back in my teens and early twenties, I wouldn't dare leave the house without a bag full of snacks. I was hungry. All. The. Time. I snacked and grazed all day long, and I made it a point to eat every few hours. I also suffered with terrible digestion and PMS. If only I knew back then what I know now—my blood sugar was irregular and I was overworking my pancreas.

THE SUGAR ROLLER COASTER

THIS IS A ROUGH DEPICTION OF WHAT HAPPENS WHEN YOU EAT SUGAR.
AFTER THE INITIAL SUGAR RUSH, YOU CRASH AND YOUR CRAVINGS INCREASE.
OTHER SYMPTOMS INCLUDE DISCOURAGING WEIGHT GAIN, FATIGUE, IRRITABILITY,
HORMONAL IMBALANCE AND DECREASED IMMUNITY.

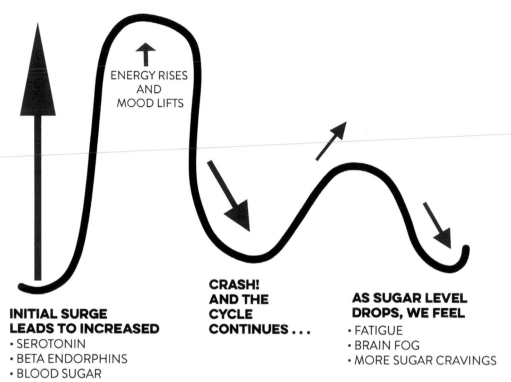

ENERGY RISES
AND
MOOD LIFTS

**INITIAL SURGE
LEADS TO INCREASED**
• SEROTONIN
• BETA ENDORPHINS
• BLOOD SUGAR

**CRASH!
AND THE
CYCLE
CONTINUES . . .**

**AS SUGAR LEVEL
DROPS, WE FEEL**
• FATIGUE
• BRAIN FOG
• MORE SUGAR CRAVINGS

It's important to note that your fat cells respond more positively to insulin if you are an athlete and you work out regularly. Athletes and people with more muscle mass can better handle eating more frequently. That's not to say they *should* be eating more frequently, but their cells are typically healthier because exercise helps with insulin sensitivity.

What about the nonathletes? What about the average, everyday woman who heads to a yoga class or goes to the gym a few times a week? Or the woman who doesn't work out at all? If you are overweight, have more than 15 pounds (6.8 kg) to lose, are obese, have PCOS, are prediabetic or diabetic, are struggling with hormonal imbalances such as PMS or irregular cycles, are constantly craving sugar, are dealing with sleep disturbances and highly stressed, well . . . you get the picture. *The 30-Day Hormone Solution* is going to help you finally shed the extra weight and get your metabolic hormones into balance so you can feel energized, healthy and vibrant.

Now, I know what you're thinking: "But Sam, I don't have diabetes, insulin resistance or issues with my blood sugar. This doesn't apply to me." The thing is, you can have normal fasting blood glucose levels but still have raging blood sugar. And to top it off, lack of sleep and high stress both have a direct impact on your insulin. Ever notice how you crave more carbs and sugar after a bad night's sleep? How many times have you told yourself you'll just reach for a healthy kale salad during a highly stressful time? I bet very rarely. That's because higher amounts of stress hormones directly impact your insulin and blood sugar levels.

Cortisol and insulin cause fat storage. If we don't get our nutrition in check, if we rely heavily on coffee, get poor-quality sleep or are stressed to the max, then we create the perfect environment for hormonal imbalances and weight gain—period. So, the next time you're choking down your veggie wrap five minutes before a meeting, consider the impact it will have on both your stress and your blood sugar levels.

THE KEYS TO BALANCING INSULIN LEVELS

What are the steps we can take to support our insulin and balance our blood sugar? I'm so glad you asked!

- **Step #1—Stop snacking.** I know this can be easier said than done, and it might take some time to get used to, but the key is to balance out your meals with protein, fat and fiber (P+F+F). This will keep you satiated, balanced and, more importantly, help you ditch those sugar cravings. The meals in your 30-Day Hormone Solution contain the perfect amount of P+F+F. Aim to eat just three meals a day, balance them appropriately and cut out the snacking.

- **Step #2—Drink 3 liters of water per day.** Typically, those with high blood glucose levels tend to be more dehydrated. Water is essential for detoxification, plus it contains zero calories—meaning it won't impact your blood sugar levels, so drink up. Staying hydrated can help your body excrete excess glucose through your urine.

- **Step #3—Choose better forms of carbohydrates.** Research published in the journal *Diabetes, Metabolic Syndrome and Obesity* suggests that monitoring carbohydrate intake is a key strategy in achieving glycemic control. It's important to choose whole food forms of carbohydrates, such as fruits and vegetables. Aim for both starchy and nonstarchy carbohydrates, with a greater focus on leafy greens, broccoli, cauliflower and cabbage, as well as starchier options such as sweet potatoes, plantains and a variety of squashes. It's important to limit your intake of sugar and white flour products. In fact, flour tends to increase insulin resistance, so choose coconut flour or almond flour instead. When limiting carbohydrates, it's important to increase your intake of protein and fat, which brings me to my next rule.

- **Step #4—Eat more protein and fat.** A 2011 study published in the *International Journal for Vitamin and Nutrition Research* found that protein consumption helped with satiety levels, energy efficiency and body composition. Protein also helps preserve both muscle and bone mass, which can often be an issue in people who have insulin resistance. As with dietary fat, the intake of monounsaturated and polyunsaturated fats was reported to improve glycemic control. Olives, olive oil, avocados, nuts and seeds are ideal choices. Omega-3-containing foods are also ideal choices for their powerful anti-inflammatory properties. Choose from hemp seeds, egg yolks, flaxseeds, chia seeds and wild-caught fish such as mackerel or sardines.

THE IMPORTANCE OF HEALTHY FATS

You'll find numerous healthy fats in your meal plan and within the recipes provided. When it comes to supplementation, one of the most important supplements I always recommend to my clients is fish oil, specifically omega-3 fatty acids from wild-caught fish. Our modern diet does not provide nearly enough of this critical nutrient as we need. It's so important to take additional omega-3s through supplementation.

Here are some reasons why omega-3s are so beneficial:

- They help switch off the genes that store fat (lipogenic) and help turn on the genes that break down fat (lipolytic).
- They can help reduce the risks of heart attack, stroke, congestive heart failure and diabetes.
- They help increase utilization of fat stores from the fat cells.
- They help reduce inflammation caused by sports and intense training.
- They help improve mental focus, memory and overall brain function. Your brain is made up of fat!
- They increase levels of serotonin, which has a very positive effect on mood.
- They lubricate your skin internally for glowing skin.
- They strengthen your hair and nails.

HIGH-QUALITY PROTEIN

Outside of healthy fats, protein is one of the most important pieces of the puzzle to help you perform at the highest level, prevent wear and tear on your muscles and joints and help balance blood sugar. Protein is essential for building and repairing muscle tissue, as well as for overall health. Optimal protein intake offers some key benefits, including:

- Support for muscle growth, strength and repair
- Enhanced recovery time between workouts
- Enhanced immune system function
- Support for fat loss
- Helps to stabilize blood sugar levels and control hunger

When it comes to protein sources, variety is key! I often see my clients eating chicken at lunch and dinner, or eggs every single day for breakfast, or using the same protein powder in their shakes for years. It's time to switch it up. Protein provides us with amino acids, which go on to support our cells, muscles, organs and tissues. To get a variety of amino acids, we need to eat a variety of proteins.

THE RIGHT CARBOHYDRATES

Where do carbs and vegetables fit into this mix? The truth is, carbohydrates often get a bad rap, but they play an important role as a source of energy and for overall health. The key is to choose the right sources of carbohydrates. You want to make sure that your blood sugar levels are stable throughout the day so that you can control your insulin levels, which helps control cravings.

When insulin is raised at the wrong time, your body will fatigue easily and store excessive amounts of fat. Here are two carbohydrate rules you should always remember as you make your way through this 30-day program:

1. Fibrous vegetables and nonstarchy carbs should be your primary source of "carbohydrate fuel" throughout the day. Fibrous carbs do not spike your blood sugar levels; this helps control cravings. You can also eat these in unlimited amounts. Think cruciferous veggies, such as broccoli, cauliflower, Brussels sprouts, asparagus and spinach.

2. Dramatically reduce the amount of grains you eat. They are not included in this program at all. If you are new to going grain-free, this is the perfect program to kick-start your grain-free journey. Back in the day, my plate was full of grains. How many of your meals do you find are centered around grains and carbs? Think about it—spaghetti and meatballs, or chicken and rice. And we can't forget sandwiches! I know many people who are packing their daily lunches with whole-wheat bread.

Speaking of wheat, did you know it can raise blood sugar levels more than white table sugar? Gluten, which is found in wheat, can cause excessive inflammation, leaky gut and heightened allergenic responses—all things we want to avoid.

TEST YOUR BLOOD SUGAR REGULARLY

When it comes to your blood sugar, if you really want to take it up a notch, I recommend purchasing a blood sugar monitor. Start testing regularly. Take your morning fasting blood sugar and your post-meal blood sugar (roughly two hours post meal). Keep a journal of your numbers along with what you are eating.

The data will be very eye-opening. I've had numerous clients find their blood sugars are incredibly high just from eating half a sweet potato. Does this mean you have to forgo sweet potatoes forever? Of course not! But it might mean that perhaps your meals aren't balanced appropriately, and it might take some time to figure out the right amount of starch you can handle in a meal. If you're feeling exhausted or tired after a meal, there's a good chance it had a direct, negative impact on your blood sugar. Outside of testing, pay attention to your symptoms and how you're feeling after eating certain foods. This can help you navigate what to include/exclude from your meals and how much starch to eat.

The following blood sugar measurements are considered healthy and normal according to the American Diabetes Association:

- If you're generally healthy, you don't have diabetes and you haven't eaten anything in the past eight hours (you've been "fasting"), it's normal for blood sugar to be between 70–99 mg/dL (less than 100 mg/dL).

- If you're healthy and you've eaten within the past two hours, it's normal for blood sugar to be anything less than 140 mg/dL.

- If you have a history of diabetes, fasting glucose should ideally be below 100 mg/dL, which might need to be managed through the use of insulin. It's also considered healthy to have levels between 70–130 mg/dL prior to eating.

- If you have diabetes and you've eaten in the past two hours, the goal is to have blood sugar below 180 mg/dL.

- If you have diabetes, you want to keep blood sugar between 100–140 mg/dL prior to bedtime and at least 100 mg/dL prior to exercising.

Having worked with many diabetics over the years in my practice, I find those measurements are still on the high side. Several studies demonstrate that fasting glucose levels should be less than 87 mg/dL. Anything above that is borderline and suggests insulin resistance. It is also most likely the cause of your fatigue, low energy, belly fat, sugar cravings and difficulty with weight loss. Blood sugar should not swing that erratically throughout the day—that is, too high in the morning, and up and down excessively throughout the course of the day. To maintain healthy weight and energy levels, you want your body to use glucose while keeping your serum blood sugar relatively stable.

I have numerous clients who have symptoms of weight gain, low energy, sleeplessness and irritability. Take my client Loraine, for example, a 40-year-old mother of two and a full-time entrepreneur. She came to me looking to lose 30 pounds (13.6 kg), could barely wake up in the morning, struggled to keep up with her kids and felt exhausted. I asked her to pay a visit to her doctor to test her fasting blood sugar levels and TSH (thyroid stimulating hormone). Her blood sugar came back at 97 mg/dL and her TSH was at 2.4. Her doctor told her she was well within the healthy range and her symptoms were just signs of being a mother and aging. How many times have you been told the same thing and sent on your way with a slew of medications?

According to the American Diabetes Association, her doctor was right. Loraine's fasting blood sugar was at a healthy range (below 100 mg/dL), but it wasn't the range I wanted to see it at. Waiting until your glucose level is above range in order to be treated is not preventive care. In fact, current guidelines have been shown to miss the diagnosis of insulin resistance in 41 to 50 percent of cases.

Loraine was not okay with accepting that her weight and fatigue were just a part of aging. She started on the 30-Day Hormone Solution and within just two weeks her fasting blood sugar stabilized between 75 and 85 mg/dL, she dropped 8 pounds (3.6 kg) and regained her energy. It's amazing what whole food nutrition can do for our hormones and health, and I can't wait for you to get started!

SUPPLEMENTATION

If you are dealing with blood sugar irregularities, insulin resistance or insulin resistant PCOS, there are many wonderful supplements that will help you get your insulin levels in check.

- **Myoinositol:** A combination of 4 g of myoinositol and 400 mcg of folic acid showed to significantly improve ovulation and conception in women with PCOS, at a rate better than 1500 mg/day of metformin.

- **Alpha-lipoic acid:** Typical dose ranges between 200 and 400 mg/day to help reduce insulin resistance.

- **Chromium picolinate:** Up to 1000 mcg/day can help improve insulin resistance.

- **Vitamin D:** This vitamin, which also functions like a hormone in the body, is essential for reducing insulin resistance. I recommend getting your levels tested so that you can dose appropriately. Typically, you want to remain on the higher end of the lab range, which can vary based on whether you live in Canada or the United States.

- **D-chiro-inositol**—At 1200 mg/day, D-chiro-inositol has been shown to improve insulin sensitivity and reduce serum testosterone levels in women with PCOS. Myoinositol (up to 4 g daily) may be substituted, or a combination of the two may be used.

BLOOD SUGAR-BALANCING BRANDS AND SUPPLEMENTS I LOVE

- Metabolic Synergy from Designs for Health
- Sensitol by Designs for Health
- Alpha-lipoic acid by Cyto-Matrix or XYMO-GEN
- Magnesium by NOW Foods, Designs for Health, Advanced Orthomolecular Research, CanPrev
- Chromium by Thorne Research, Advanced Orthomolecular Research or NFH
- Chromium Synergy by Designs for Health
- D-chiro-inositol or myoinositol by Advanced Orthomolecular Research, Designs for Health or NFH
- Vitamin D liquid by Designs for Health, Advanced Orthomolecular Research or CanPrev

PART 2:

FOUNDATIONS OF THE 30-DAY HORMONE SOLUTION

CHAPTER 5:
MASTERING YOUR HORMONE MIND-SET:
WHY "I'LL START ON MONDAY" MEANS YOU'VE ALREADY FAILED

After fifteen years of coaching women, I've learned a thing or two when it comes to achieving your health goals. The biggest predictor of success is your mind-set. It's time for a bit of butt-kicking with a side of love. If you have big and lofty goals you want to achieve for yourself, whether it be with your health or your life, you have got to listen up.

I can't tell you the number of times I've been in conversations with women and they spend the entire time complaining about their symptoms and share with me intimate details about their struggles—from not wanting to be seen naked in front of their partner to avoiding family gatherings, picnics at the beach or vacations altogether—on top of the physical symptoms of bloating, exhaustion, weight gain and joint pain, just to name a few.

This is no way to live. Period.

Transformation is not linear. Your health, wellness and healing require a deep commitment and patience. Diving in also requires an understanding that things *will* go wrong. The scale won't *always* budge. The pain might come back. But this doesn't mean you give up and stop trying. It just means you tweak where you are and keep moving forward.

I often ask my clients, "Are you committed to your current circumstance or to the possibility of your future?" In fact, many of the women I coach can't even comprehend what their future self could look and feel like.

And so, the first step is to sit quietly with your journal and start to write out WHO YOU ARE in the future. What do you feel? How do you look? What are you doing? As you do this exercise, I really want you to think about what's possible for your health. If you committed 100 percent of your time and energy and love to healing, what would the outcome look like? Write about that.

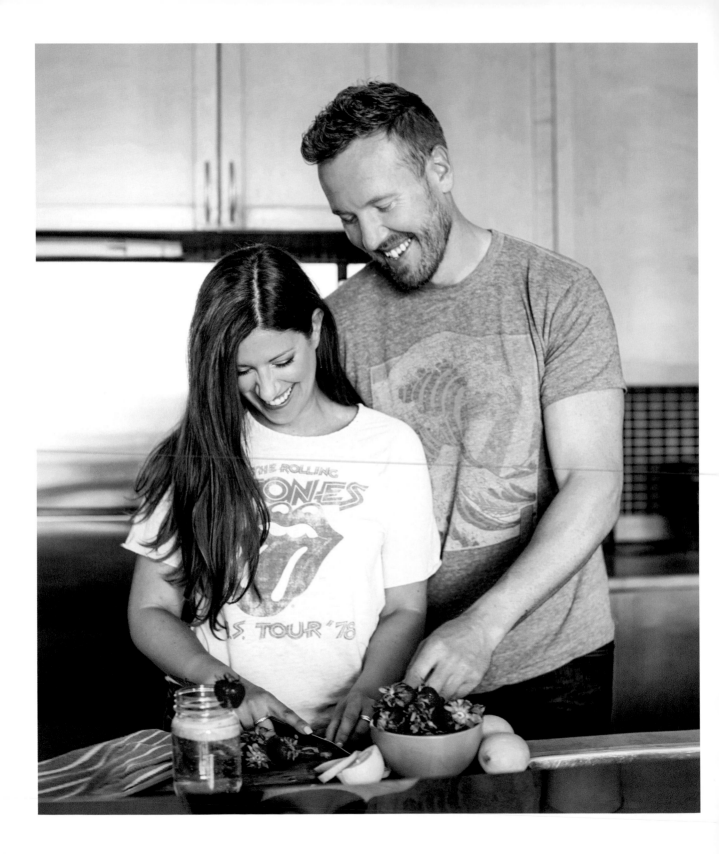

Next, spend time writing about what would happen if you committed to your current circumstance. If you stay the same and do nothing, then what? Are you willing to spend another five, ten, twenty, thirty years feeling and looking this way? I can bet the answer is no.

Wherever you are on your health journey, you must do the uncomfortable work. Dive in and begin right where you are. There is no right time to begin. Beginning starts now, taking imperfect action and knowing that your journey will get messy along the way. And that is okay, my friend. You are human, after all. How many times have you said to yourself, "I'll start on Monday"? This type of mentality is failure mentality. Failure to recognize that you have the power within you right now to make a choice that supports your future self and supports the health and healing you so deeply long for.

Our diet dilemma has everything to do with food, and nothing to do with food. Yes, the food matters. It affects how we feel and impacts our overall health. But it goes beyond the food on our plate. This is where the mind-set piece comes in, and it's the one area most of us don't want to address.

Many of the women I've coached are living in fear. Fear of the scale. Fear of the visit to the doctor. Fear of the changing room mirror. Fear of spending money on themselves. Fear of what others might think. Bottom line: it boils down to fear. And the more we fear, the more we tend to retreat and resort to destructive habits.

It's key to find a community of people you can trust who will hold you accountable. Sharing your fears and insecurities with others is essential in helping you reach your health goals. This is why having a coach is so important. Having someone who can provide you with the right plan, the right system and support and accountability will help you get to your goals a lot faster. As a coach, I stand for the possibility of my clients and I provide the path and support they need, helping them understand their fears, work through their fears and step more into their personal power.

I've used food as the vehicle to help women achieve more powerful, holistic, purpose-driven lives because I know firsthand what whole foods can do for your health and body. To succeed at losing weight, balancing hormones and healing your body, you have to take responsibility for your actions. *You* are in control. *You* have the power.

This can often be scary because knowing that it's all on you, that your destiny is in your hands, is a lot of pressure. But it's also the truth. We have to take radical responsibility for how we show up for ourselves, for how we treat ourselves and for what we choose to put on our plates. Ultimately, it's your choice and you're the only one in control of that.

It's very easy to believe that some magic pill, shake, detox kit or diet is going to be the key to your success. The solution to your healing won't be found in the bottom of some pill bottle. It's you. And the only way to move forward from where you are now, to where you desire to go, is to make uncomfortable and difficult choices. That is all. One difficult choice after another. Choosing *better* for yourself and letting go of your comfort zone. I acknowledge you for being here, for reading this book and for taking the uncomfortable leap forward toward a more powerful and healthy future.

To get your mind-set in tip-top shape, let's map out some simple strategies so you can get clear on your journey ahead.

#1: UNDERSTAND THE BIG PICTURE

I shared above how the first step is to journal about who you are in the future. Another way to look at this is to determine what your "WHY" is. Why did you pick up this book? What is it that you are trying to transform and how long have you been trying? And girl, you gotta go deep. I don't want to hear, "I just want to eat better." Purpose drives us, so spend the time to dig in and get clear on the big picture.

Connect your why to your daily decisions, the foods you choose to eat and the way you choose to live. This is not about shaming ourselves or feeling bad about our choices. But let's get real. Who are you trying to please? What are you avoiding in your life by sitting down in front of Netflix with a bowl of ice cream?

I work with many women in my practice who are running at hyperspeed, filling up their calendars and busy with family and kids. In the mix of it all, they are gaining weight, feeling frumpy and exhausted and losing their zest for life. All that busy-ness is detaching them from themselves—from who they are at the core and what they long for. And over time, this becomes their norm. They put themselves last and they lose touch with their real authentic selves. But more importantly, they lose touch with those around them. They can't show up for their kids or their husband and so, they bury themselves in the fridge, the glass of wine or the bar of chocolate. Get honest with yourself and journal your why.

#2: SET GOALS

Let's talk about goal setting. I want you to set a realistic goal for yourself. Remember, this isn't a race. If weight loss is a goal, keep in mind how long it took to come on and be realistic with the amount of time it will take to come off. Losing 30 pounds (13.6 kg) in 30 days is not realistic, and a goal like that will only set you up for failure. The problem with "diets" is that you've most likely been on one in the past and it worked, until it didn't! What I mean by this is that your past diet failures are still hanging out in your brain. There is a voice in your head feeling unsure of how exactly to move forward because ultimately you think it won't work.

The only thing that won't work is you and not trying. So, pick yourself up, dust yourself off and take a deep breath. Forgive yourself for whatever diet program you've done in the past and move forward. Press delete, send that old way of thinking to the trash and begin anew.

Your goals must be simple, attainable and realistic. They should also reflect more than just your weight. We often minimize the small successes: prepping our food, drinking more water, taking our daily supplements, going to bed on time and moving our bodies. These are successes that should not be forgotten or minimized.

For optimal success, spend time mapping out your week and schedule. Get clear on when you can prep food. Who can you ask for help? What will you measure beyond your weight? What is a realistic time frame for achieving your goals? And given your current circumstances and lifestyle, are you setting realistic goals or aiming *just* a little too high?

It's crazy how some women will enroll in my programs and in 30 days I'll hear how they are sleeping better and have more energy; their skin cleared up; they don't feel as bloated; they feel happier and the brain fog has lifted. *BUT*, the scale barely moved so they won't be continuing to implement the program. *SAY WHAT??* That is crazy talk. Banking all your success on the scale will only leave you feeling defeated. The scale does not take into account sodium or water retention or your hormonal fluctuations. It will not always be precise. I suggest you track your measurements every 1 to 2 weeks, and only weigh yourself once a week, if that. And ladies, don't weigh yourself or go skinny jean shopping around your period. Okay?

#3: MAKE POWERFUL CHOICES

You are not on or off, you just ARE. The typical diet mentality is that you're only ever on a diet or off a diet. This is why one glass of wine sends you back into "I screwed up and I am giving up" mode. Are you ready to give up being a perfectionist and accept being a human BEING and not a human DOING?

Let me say this loud and clear—there are no screw-ups. Every day you have the opportunity to be better and make powerful choices. It doesn't matter if your day got off to a rocky start and you ate the muffin. You have the opportunity at your next meal to get back on track and move forward. It's all good.

Achieving your health goals will not be linear. There will be ups and downs, so the sooner you can accept this, the sooner you can move on and take powerful action toward your goals. And speaking of action, when you find yourself slipping, unprepped, overworked, stressed out and falling into those old unhealthy habits, just take one positive action in the direction of your goal. This will help to reinforce that you are in control. This might look like a walk around your office, drinking a large glass of water or calling a friend to have a chat. Bottom line, interrupt your cycle by taking action.

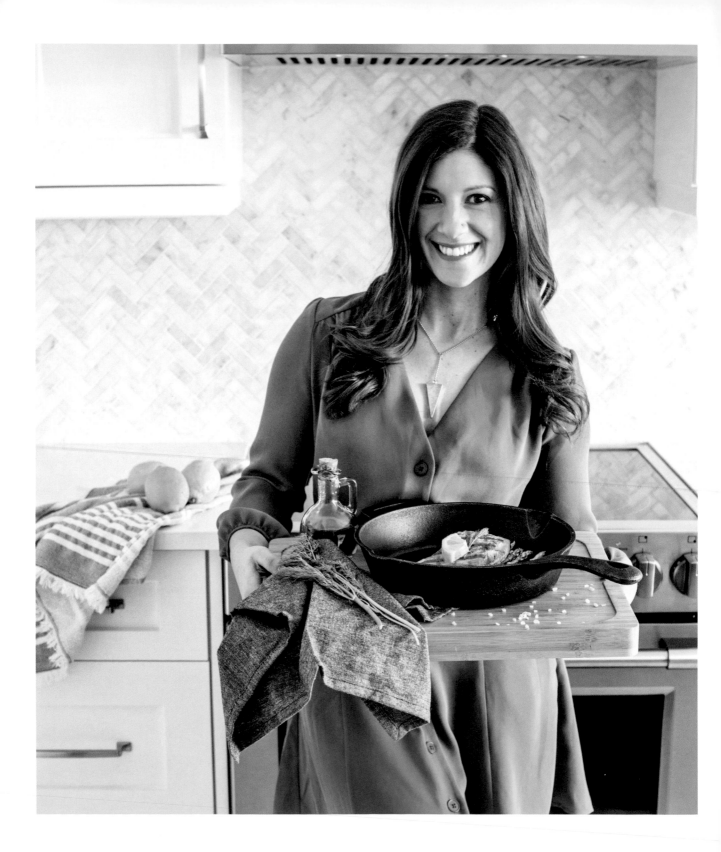

CHAPTER 6:

THE PALEO APPROACH TO BALANCING AND RESETTING HORMONES

If you want to set yourself up for success and achieve your health and hormone goals, it starts in your kitchen with high-quality food. It is essential to clean out the foods that are wreaking havoc on your hormones—goodbye sugary treats! Nothing is worse than a whole week of clean eating, exercising and the right mind-set suddenly ruined by opening up your cupboards to find that chocolate-covered peanut bar. You know what I mean!

In the past, I followed a vegan diet, vegetarian diet, macrobiotic and . . . well, you name it, I tried it. Back in 2013, I started to experience digestive issues, such as bloating and terrible stomach pains. I wasn't sure what was going on, so I went for a food intolerance test. Sure enough, the foods I was eating the most—bananas, avocados, beans and legumes—were causing me to react to them.

I eliminated these foods from my diet, and I worked on healing my gut so that, at some point, I could bring these foods back into my diet with fewer issues. This was when I decided to reintroduce meat back into my diet. I hadn't eaten a steak in years, and it was not something I was really excited about, even still to this day. But I do remember being out for dinner at a steakhouse and I decided to go for it. I will never forget that meal. The steak was perfectly cooked, incredibly juicy and delicious. I literally felt creatine and B_{12} coursing through my veins. It was a wild experience, and it led me on a deeper path to discover the Paleo diet. Even though I had read *The Paleo Diet* by Loren Cordain back in my early twenties, it just didn't sink in at the time.

REAL TALK

When it comes to diets, it is essential that you find what works for you. I can share from my own experience, and the experiences of the thousands of women I've coached over the years, that eliminating grains, beans, gluten, dairy and sugar has had a profound impact on my health.

My health and my lab work improved once I started to introduce more animal proteins and quality fats and I gave up gluten and grains. This doesn't mean I never eat grains or beans. I tune into what my body wants, and sometimes I want to eat a taco bowl with a serving of white rice. Other times, I want a bean soup or feel like diving into a massive plate of hummus. These aren't staples in my diet, and if I feel like having them every now and again, I do.

With that said, if you haven't cut out grains and beans before, I highly suggest taking the 30-Day Hormone Solution for a test-drive and see how you feel. Afterward, go ahead and add them back in, paying attention to symptoms that might arise. There is a lot of trial and error when it comes to nutrition; we are all so bio-individual, and what works for one person does not work for another.

I am often asked about my thoughts on the Keto diet or the carnivore diet. Depending on your specific health and needs, these diets may benefit you. In fact, I often encourage a higher fat intake, as I find most women avoid eating fat. In my 12-week Metabolic Reset online weight loss program we focus on a higher fat and lower carb intake.

BUT, before jumping on diet bandwagons, start with your foundation FIRST. Let this program be the gateway to cleaning up your diet, understanding your body and hormones and eliminating inflammatory foods. From there you'll have a deeper understanding of your health and needs, and you can make the appropriate tweaks and modifications.

Be gentle with yourself. Go slow. Have the courage to cut out certain foods so you can truly assess how your body feels without them. Tune in. Pay attention and honor your body where it's at right now.

WHAT YOU WILL BE EATING

What will you be eating on the 30-Day Hormone Solution plan? Let's take a look at your delicious options.

- **Organic, Pasture-Raised, Grass-Fed Animal Products.** I emphasize organic and pasture-raised, but I understand that this is not always feasible. Compared to conventional animal products, organic animal meats will not contain GMOs, pesticides, antibiotics and harmful hormones. Choose from beef, chicken, lamb, venison, pork, duck, turkey and even liver and organ meats as well as eggs. Otherwise, be sure to look for hormone-free and antibiotic-free meats when shopping.

- **Wild-Caught Fish.** Salmon, mackerel, sardines and anchovies are all great sources of high-quality omega-3s that are anti-inflammatory and heart protective.

- **Starchy Vegetables.** Choose from plantains, sweet potatoes, squashes, yucca and yams. They are loaded with vitamins and minerals, and they're great substitutes for grains.

- **Nonstarchy Vegetables.** Choose cruciferous vegetables such as broccoli, cauliflower, Brussels sprouts, and choose leafy greens such as kale, spinach and Swiss chard. Head to ewg.org and search for the Clean 15 and Dirty Dozen lists. These provide you with updated lists of the foods to purchase organic and the foods that contain higher amounts of herbicides and pesticides.

- **Fermented Foods.** Include sauerkraut, kimchi, low-sugar kombucha and coconut kefir for their gut-supportive probiotics.

- **Fruits.** Aim for lower-glycemic fruits such as apples and pears. Also choose raspberries, blueberries, strawberries and cherries. Aim for no more than three servings of fruit a day, including it as part of your meal and not as a snack. More on that in Chapter 9, page 92.

- **Healthy Fats.** Choose from saturated, monounsaturated and polyunsaturated fats, such as coconut oil, grass-fed butter, ghee, olive oil, avocado oil, fish oil and flaxseed oil. This also includes olives, avocados, nuts and seeds. Keep in mind that animal products also contain saturated fat and using animal fats, such as duck fat, beef tallow and lard, is also acceptable.

- **Herbs and Spices.** Using a blend of herbs and spices can add so much flavor to your meals. Choose high-quality sea salt, such as Redmond Real Salt, and choose from a variety of fresh and dried herbs. You'll notice that in many of my recipes I do not include black pepper. By all means, feel free to add this, but I choose to leave it out because many people can be quite intolerant to it. Some of my favorite herb and spice brands include Primal Palate, Simply Organic, Bragg, Frontier, Herbamare and Cha's Organics.

- **Condiments.** Include balsamic vinegar, apple cider vinegar, coconut aminos, mayonnaise, ketchup and Dijon mustard. These are all fine during your reset and beyond, but do keep in mind that many brands add sugar and preservatives to their ingredients list. Be sure to read your labels and opt for quality brands. I personally like Primal Kitchen, and if you're using fish sauce, Red Boat is gluten-free.

WHAT YOU WON'T BE EATING

The truth is that cleaning out your cupboards takes courage. It takes courage to let go of all the foods that are near and dear to you, foods that are truly sucking the life out of you and holding you back from achieving the health and vitality you desire. We have such a deep emotional connection to our food, and throwing it out can often be quite hard.

Open your cupboards and take a look at the foods that are no longing serving you. Keep in mind, you can donate nonperishable food items to charities or your local food bank. Your cupboards might start to look empty, but you'll be replacing all the low-quality foods with clean, healthy and organic goodness.

WHAT TO SWAP

- **Canned vegetables or fruit:** Replace these with fresh vegetables and fruit.

- **Fruit juices:** Swap out fruit juices with a green veggie juice or smoothie that you can make at home.

- **White pasta/breads:** Replace pasta and gluten-containing breads with quality carbohydrate sources, such as sweet potatoes, butternut squash, spaghetti squash, yams and other starchy and fibrous vegetables.

- **Low-fat/high-sugar treats:** Swap these for homemade treats made with quality gluten-free and grain-free flours, better-quality sugar and hormone-healthy fats. Head to page 204 for delicious dessert and treat options.

- **Diet drinks:** Swap these for fresh spring-water, coconut water, kombucha, fresh smoothies and green juices.

WHY DO WE NEED TO DITCH THESE FOODS ANYWAY?

We need to ditch packaged, fake foods that contain little to no nutritional value. Most canned foods are highly salted and contain a variety of preservatives. Plus, they are stored in a can with a BPA lining and other potential toxic chemicals that are leeching into your food. If you are vegetarian and choose to eat beans and legumes from the can, I highly recommend Eden Organic products. All their cans are BPA-free, plus they use kombu, a sea vegetable, to add salt to their beans. They are a great company that sources quality, organic ingredients.

Fruit juices can be a tough one, especially if you have kids. The fact is, fruit juice is just sugar. There are no nutrients, minerals or essential vitamins in a juice box that you can't get from simply eating the whole fruit. The whole fruit will provide your body with vitamins, fiber and other essential phytonutrients. With the rise in child obesity and diabetes, I would caution the use or overuse of fruit juices.

THE PROBLEM WITH GLUTEN

What's the deal with gluten? Gluten is a protein found in wheat and other grains such as barley, rye, oats and spelt. It acts like a glue. It has a binding capability that can cause issues within the gastrointestinal tract.

Wheat is not what it once was. It's the hybridized wheat that has become a problem: it has undergone mutations; its genetics have been altered; and it has been exposed to numerous chemicals.

FOODS TO SWAP

FOOD		SWAP WITH
CANNED VEGETABLES OR FRUIT	→	REPLACE WITH FRESH VEGETABLES AND FRUIT.
FRUIT JUICES	→	REPLACE WITH A GREEN VEGGIE JUICE OR SMOOTHIE THAT YOU CAN MAKE AT HOME.
WHITE PASTA/BREADS	→	REPLACE WITH QUALITY CARBOHYDRATE SOURCES, SUCH AS SWEET POTATOES, BUTTERNUT SQUASH, SPAGHETTI SQUASH, YAMS AND OTHER STARCHY AND FIBROUS VEGETABLES.
LOW-FAT/HIGH-SUGAR TREATS	→	REPLACE WITH HOMEMADE TREATS MADE WITH QUALITY GLUTEN-FREE AND GRAIN-FREE FLOURS, BETTER-QUALITY SUGAR AND HORMONE-HEALTHY FATS.
DIET DRINKS	→	REPLACE WITH FRESH SPRINGWATER, COCONUT WATER, KOMBUCHA, FRESH SMOOTHIES AND GREEN JUICES.

It may look the same, but it's wearing a sneaky disguise, and we welcome it onto our plates daily, in many different forms: whole-wheat, seven-grain and multigrain bread; cinnamon raisin bagels; hamburger and hot dog buns; French bread and pita bread; soft pretzels; pancakes, waffles and cereals; baked goods; pasta, egg noodles and lasagna noodles; and even condiments. Almost all processed food contains gluten, as it is commonly used as a thickening agent, binder or flavoring agent (as a malt).

A great way to remember which grains contain gluten is by using the acronym BROWS, which stands for Barley, Rye, Oats, Wheat and Spelt. This will come in handy when cruising the grocery aisle!

But going gluten-free isn't always the answer. Swapping out all your pastas, breads and bagels for gluten-free options does not mean you are making a healthier choice. Many gluten-free products contain starches, preservatives and an unnecessary amount of added sugars. Be cautious about the brands you buy, and always read your labels. Bake up my Grain-Free Almond Flour Bread recipe on page 100, and I promise you won't be missing your morning slice of white bread.

WHY NO GRAINS?

Between the USDA Food Pyramid and Canada's Food Guide (which has just recently been updated, thank God!), we are told that grains should make up the base of our diets. Where do you think this advice has gotten us? Obesity and diabetes are on the rise, with diabetes showing up in young children and teenagers.

Grains are processed, high-carbohydrate foods that break down into sugar in your body. They have the ability to cause fatigue and unstable blood sugar levels, especially in carb- and sugar-sensitive individuals. Grains also contain certain antinutrients that block the absorption of minerals and other nutrients. The protein portion of grains is covered in a sticky substance called lectin that contributes to inflammation in the digestive tract.

Grains include wheat, rye, spelt, bulgur, corn, semolina, triticale, durum, oats, couscous, rice, quinoa, millet, bulgur, buckwheat and amaranth. Examples of refined grain-based foods are granola, cereal, bread, bagels, muffins, scones, cookies, baked goods, croissants, English muffins, flour tortillas, pancakes, waffles, pasta, brown rice pasta, pita bread and more. To support and optimize gut function, grains are eliminated on a Paleo diet.

LEGUMES

Like grains, legumes are high-carbohydrate foods that contain lectins. Many people have difficulty digesting legumes, often leading to fatigue, bloating and blood sugar instability. Legumes include all beans, except green beans: black beans, white beans, butter beans, lima beans, adzuki beans, pinto beans, navy beans, garbanzo beans and kidney beans, as well as lentils and soybeans.

Beans and legumes contain a chemical called phytic acid. Phytic acid is a compound that comes from the phosphorus found in plants. Too much phytic acid can inhibit the thyroid, hamper digestion and leach vital minerals, such as zinc and iron, from the body. Phytic acid also interferes with the natural enzymes your body needs to digest your food.

Overconsumption of phytic acid is actually a big source of digestive upset for many people. Legumes are not a part of your 30-Day Hormone Solution, but you can reintroduce them back into your diet after your reset and assess for any symptoms that may arise.

DAIRY

I have a weakness for dairy—mainly cheese! Although I cut out cow's milk dairy many years ago, I will include some goat or sheep's milk feta in my diet every now and again. Dairy products include milk, cream, yogurt, kefir, cheese, cottage cheese, ice cream, gelato, frozen yogurt and the list goes on and on.

Lactose intolerance is common, and it often goes unnoticed. Many people only discover that they respond poorly to dairy products once they've removed them, because they find the symptoms of lactose intolerance tend to be quite clearly relieved on a dairy-free diet. For many people, the A1 casein in cow's milk—primarily Holstein and Friesian cows—is highly inflammatory. Milk that has predominately A2 casein tends to be less of an issue; this comes from dairy cows in Africa, Asia, Western Europe and North America.

A1 casein can be quite problematic for type 1 diabetics, and it is highly implicated in autoimmune disease. A1 casein forms a powerful inflammatory opiate in the body called casomorphin. This can contribute to lymphatic congestion, weight gain, mood disorders, acne, eczema, upper respiratory infections and asthma.

If you can relate to any of these issues, I suggest eliminating dairy for a full 30 days, then reintroduce it back into your diet and pay attention to the symptoms that show up. Many people can tolerate unpasteurized or raw dairy products because they contain the enzymes that help the body digest dairy, and these enzymes are killed during the high-heat pasteurization process.

"DIET" DRINKS

What about low-fat and sugar-free "diet" drinks? Unfortunately, these are just a huge marketing ploy to draw you in, tricking you into thinking you're doing something good for your heart and your waistline. "Low fat" typically means more sugar has been added to a product, and "diet" typically means that a no-calorie artificial sweetener has been added.

Diet sodas are doing nothing to support your health and hormones. In fact, a study in the journal *Stroke* showed that people who drank at least one diet soda a day were three times as likely to have a stroke or develop dementia as those who avoided these beverages. Artificial sweeteners are neurotoxic—they can actually alter and destroy brain cells. Ditch them, and your brain and your body will thank you.

SUGARS

Indulging in something sweet is bound to happen. I mean, c'mon, we're human, after all. A little bit of sweetness in our lives keeps us sane.

But there is definitely a difference between good sugar and bad sugar. This doesn't mean that you can eat all the "good" sugar that your little heart desires. And I promise you'll love the dessert and treat recipes I've included in this book, and they won't spike your blood sugar the way most traditional desserts will.

Here is a list of sugars and artificial sweeteners to avoid:

- Table sugar
- High fructose corn syrup
- Sucrose
- Maltodextrin
- Fructose
- Sweet'N Low
- Equal
- Splenda
- Sugar Twin
- NutraSweet
- Acesulfame potassium (Ace K)

Swap these artificial sugars with natural options, but do keep in mind that sugar is still sugar. Overdoing it will cause your blood sugar to go haywire and lead to other hormonal imbalances. Keep your intake minimal.

- **Stevia:** This plant sugar comes from the sunflower family and is a no-calorie sweetener. It's great for baking and in coffee or tea. Some people find it to be quite bitter, so be sure to taste-test to your preference.

- **Raw Honey:** Raw honey is antibacterial and great for immunity, plus it's amazing for soothing a sore throat. I love Beekeeper's Naturals brand.

- **Coconut Sugar:** This sugar comes from the coconut sap. It is low on the glycemic index, meaning it does not spike blood sugar the way regular sugar does.

- **Organic Maple Syrup:** A favorite on pancakes, maple syrup is loaded with B vitamins and minerals.

- **Monk Fruit:** This is the sugar I use in most of my baking recipes. It is also called *luo han guo*. It looks like a small gourd and grows on a vine. Many monk fruit brands contain erythritol, which some people may react to. Be sure to read ingredient labels when purchasing monk fruit if you want to avoid erythritol. I use the brand Lakanto, which does contain erythritol, with no issues. Also check out Julian Bakery, which is free of erythritol.

There are many ways to add sweetness to your life without relying on high-sugar treats and desserts. Here are a few ideas:

- Protein balls made with stevia or dried superfoods, such as goji berries
- Low-glycemic fruits, such as green apples, berries and grapefruit
- Smoothies made with natural low-glycemic fruits, such as blueberries
- Baked apples with cinnamon
- Celery sticks with almond butter and cinnamon
- Shredded coconut with pumpkin seeds and raw cacao nibs
- Baked sweet potato with ghee, coconut oil or olive oil and cinnamon

It's also important to look at other ways to add sweetness in your life, incorporating more self-care and optimizing your well-being. If you find you are having a hard time giving up sugar, the 30-Day Hormone Solution is going to help you combat that! Other strategies to include are meditation, yoga or tai chi, exercise, dancing, being in nature, taking a bath or sauna, dry skin brushing, talking with friends and laughter.

THE ESSENTIALS

WE TEND TO OVERTHINK AND OVERDO WHEN IT COMES TO OUR HEALTH. WE ARE QUICK TO SELF-DIAGNOSE, THINK WE NEED TO INVEST IN EXPENSIVE TESTING AND OFTEN FORGET ABOUT THE ESSENTIALS. IF YOU FEEL LIKE CRAP, WORKING WITH A PRACTITIONER TO HELP YOU UNCOVER WHAT'S GOING ON AND GETTING YOUR HORMONES TESTED IS AN INCREDIBLE STEP IN THE RIGHT DIRECTION TOWARD HEALING. HOWEVER, HAVE YOU COVERED THE ESSENTIALS? HERE ARE SOME IMPORTANT QUESTIONS TO ASK YOURSELF WHEN YOU FEEL LIKE YOUR HEALTH HAS TAKEN A TURN FOR THE WORSE.

#1	**AM I EATING A NUTRITIOUS, WHOLE FOODS DIET AND EATING IN MEALS, NOT SNACKS?**
#2	**AM I GETTING ENOUGH QUALITY SLEEP? AM I WELL RESTED?**
#3	**AM I HYDRATED ENOUGH, DRINKING AT LEAST 3 LITERS OF WATER A DAY?**
#4	**AM I STRESSED AND ANXIOUS AND NOT MANAGING MY DAILY STRESSORS WELL? AM I BEING AN ACTOR IN MY LIFE OR A REACTOR?**
#5	**AM I MOVING MY BODY AND SWEATING AT LEAST THREE OR FOUR DAYS A WEEK?**
#6	**AM I GOING OUTSIDE AND EXPOSING MYSELF TO THE SUN AND BREATHING IN FRESH AIR?**

WE OFTEN OVERLOOK THESE ESSENTIALS BECAUSE THEY ARE SO EASY TO IMPLEMENT THAT WE FORGET HOW POWERFUL THEY TRULY ARE!

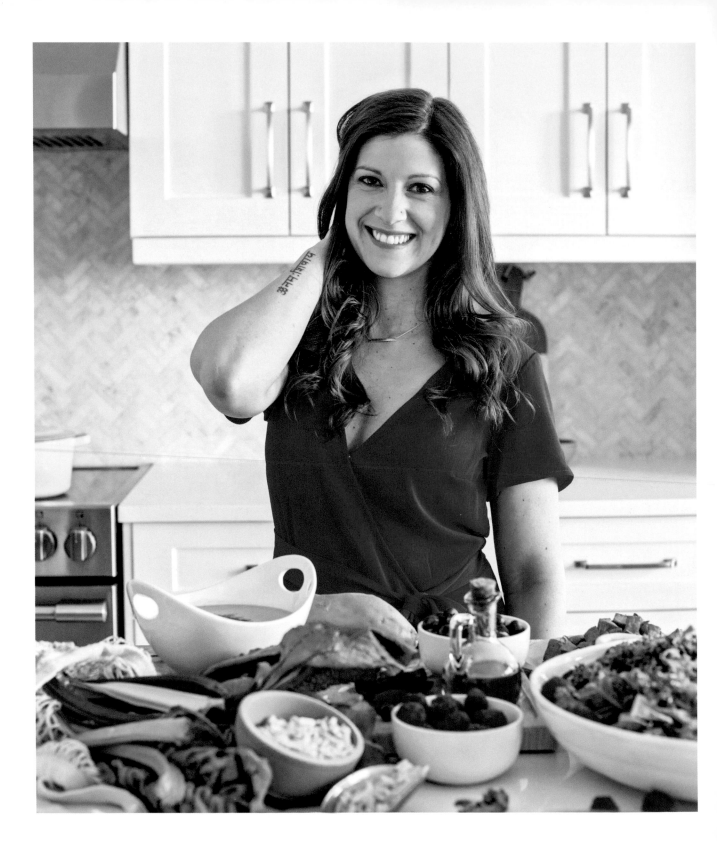

CHAPTER 7:
SLEEP, HYDRATION AND DETOX:
SOLUTION ESSENTIALS

SLEEP

When it comes to weight loss and balancing hormones, we are often quick to jump onto the next fad diet. Or we buy the latest supplement or fancy shake. It's easy to forget about the foundational things that drastically improve our health, with sleep being at the top of that list. *If you're not sleeping, you're not healing.* Quality sleep is essential to our health, and that is why it's a reset essential.

Back in my university days I was bartending four or five nights of the week. How else do you think I paid for university?! Sure, in our twenties we are more resilient and can bounce back from lack of sleep, but that doesn't mean it's a good thing or something we should take advantage of.

Going to school full-time and bartending from 5 p.m. until 3 a.m. most nights was crazy! Talk about adrenal fatigue. Those late nights turned me into a night owl. I would stay up late watching TV, reading or organizing my closet—no joke. The worst part was the later I stayed up, the later I would eat. I remember getting home from the bar at 4 a.m. and raiding the fridge for food. Then I'd hop into bed on a full tummy. This was a terrible idea. Those late nights carried on for years, and 2 to 4 a.m. bedtimes and 10 a.m. wake-ups left me lethargic.

When I started working full-time, I had no choice but to change my sleeping habits. I had to be up at 7 a.m. and my 2 a.m. bedtime needed to change . . . ASAP!

What I needed was to create a nighttime ritual, and I encourage you do the same for yourself. Our bodies crave routine. In fact, we are very connected to the sun and moon, which is why our hormones, specifically cortisol and melatonin, mimic the rhythms of light and dark.

When the sun rises, our cortisol is at its highest, allowing us to rise out of bed and have the energy to perform our daily tasks. As the sun sets and the moon rises, our cortisol levels drop, allowing us to slow down, relax and get ready for sleep. Melatonin begins its real work at night, when the sun sets. Melatonin is like your body's internal clock. It's a powerful hormone and antioxidant, and it allows you to get into a deep slumber.

OPTIMIZE YOUR SLEEP WHILE YOU'RE AWAKE

Quality sleep isn't just dependent on what you do at night. What you do during the day counts just as much. In order to improve your melatonin, you must expose yourself to enough sunlight during the day. The exposure to wide-spectrum light allows your body to produce sufficient serotonin; this, in turn, will help you produce sufficient melatonin at night.

Most people wake up, eat breakfast, get in the car and head to work, where they spend eight or more hours of their day under artificial light. Then they get back in the car and head home with barely any outdoor exposure.

Artificial light—any indoor light—will provide roughly 500 to possibly 5000 LUX light. Outdoor sun exposure, even on a cloudy day, can provide 10,000 to roughly 25,000 LUX light. That's a huge difference. Blue light, in particular from your computer screen, TV screen or phone, has a direct impact on lowering melatonin levels.

Bottom line: Just like we want to avoid junk food, we want to avoid junk light. I suggest wearing blue-blocking glasses while at work or on your computer and even while watching TV. This will have a profound impact on your hormones and sleep quality.

I've made it a point to go outside first thing in the morning for a walk to expose myself to an abundance of LUX light. After just one week of morning walks, both my deep sleep and my REM levels improved greatly—which I tracked with my Oura Ring sleep tracker. If morning walks are not an option for you, I suggest investing in a light therapy box or turning on your lights as bright as you can first thing in the morning.

This brings to me an important point, and that is *recess*. Remember recess in elementary school? Heading outside to play with your friends, run around and spend time in nature? As adults, we are missing this. Time in the sun, connection with the earth and nature, playing, running and breathing in fresh air is no longer a part of our daily routines. Instead, we've traded our recess days for a coffee and cigarette break.

Make recess a priority in your life. This connection to the earth and sun will provide you healing energy and improve your sleep.

TOP TIPS FOR HAVING THE BEST SLEEP EVER

1. **Eat your last meal at least two to three hours before bed to allow yourself enough time to digest your food effectively.** This meal should consist of a quality protein source, green leafy and/or nonstarchy vegetables, and quality fat. If you find yourself having a hard time falling asleep, include a starchy vegetable, such as a sweet potato, with your dinner and see if that helps.

2. **Turn the lights down low.** Real low. Bright light will affect melatonin production, your sleepy hormone. Melatonin helps you sleep and begins its work in the evening. Artificial light will affect how well you naturally produce melatonin. Dim the lights, light candles and create a sensual environment that allows your body to wind down. This means no computer or TV light at least an hour before going to bed! Limiting your exposure to artificial light after the sun sets will improve your sleep dramatically.

3. **Overhaul your bedroom.** Create a space that is conducive for sleep. NO phone. NO office work. NO bright lighting—even the light on your alarm clock is bad news. Be conscious of chemicals in your bedroom. Be conscious of the laundry detergent you use to wash your sheets or, better yet, how frequently you wash your sheets and rid them of bacteria. And speaking of sheets . . . I recommend organic cotton.

4. **Soak in the tub.** A warm bath with Epsom salts is a great way to unwind before bed. Epsom salts contain magnesium, which is an important mineral that aids muscle soreness and stiffness, reduces aches and pains, and allows your body to relax.

5. **Avoid stimulants.** Light is a stimulant at night, but so is your coffee. Make sure to have your coffee before 2 p.m. so that you give your body sufficient time to utilize the caffeine. If you find you are sensitive to caffeine, green tea may also be just as stimulating, as it contains naturally occurring caffeine.

6. **Have sex.** This is a great way to unwind before bed. Sex helps reduce stress by producing feel-good hormones, such as oxytocin. In fact, oxytocin helps lower your cortisol levels (the stress hormone), which means a deeper and more relaxed sleep for you my friend! Oxytocin is also known as the "love" hormone. This "love" hormone can help build a deeper connection between you and your partner.

7. **Get to bed before 11 p.m. to optimize your hormones.** Melatonin is at its peak level between 11 p.m. and 3 a.m. This means no lights at that time, even if you wake up to go pee!

8. **Wear blue-blocking glasses during the day while at your computer.** I have a yellow pair that are for computer work. I also have a red pair that are more heavy duty and specific for sleep, so I wear them about an hour before bed if I'm watching TV. I also advise downloading the free app called f.lux (justgetflux .com). This software will automatically change the tint of your computer screen based on the sun rising and setting to help mimic natural light rhythms.

9. **Reduce your sugar consumption and maintain consistent blood sugar levels.** Adrenaline can wake you up in the middle of the night if you have significant blood sugar fluctuations, and the body will often secrete adrenaline in response to blood sugar lows.

10. **Move your body.** Getting in some regular exercise will help support blood sugar, maintain healthy muscle mass and bone density, and support overall health. Our metabolism gets lazy by sitting all day. In turn, we also experience more fatigue and brain fog. Simply standing at your desk versus sitting all day will help keep your energy levels up during the day and make you sleepier during nighttime hours.

Implement a digital detox. I suggest you stop sleeping with the enemy! I'm referring to your cell phone, that is. Get your phone out of the bedroom. If you are using it as your alarm, find another alarm. The electromagnetic frequency (EMF) emitting from your phone is so strong that it can impair how your body handles and deals with stress.

I love how Dr. Mercola describes the impact that EMFs have on our body. He explains that our body is a complex communication device where cells, tissues, organs and organisms all "talk" to each other. At each of these levels, the communication includes finely tuned bio-electrical transmitters and receivers, which are tuned like tuning into a radio station. What happens when you expose a radio antenna to a significant amount of external noise? You get static from the noise and that is what is happening to your body in today's electro-smog environment. Imagine that? The communication happening between your cells, tissues, organs and even hormones is disrupted simply by talking on your cell phone, sitting in your Wi-Fi office or walking outside in the city. This is just another reason why getting outside in nature is so essential—it helps cleanse and detox your body from EMFs.

Limit your exposure as much as you can to EMFs. Be conscious of how frequently you use your phone, how often you hold it in your hand and whether you choose to keep it by your bedside. Sleep is so important for our overall health, so be sure to create a relaxing environment that will aid in the best sleep ever. You *must* make sleep a priority if you're looking to improve your hormonal health. It's a nonnegotiable.

HYDRATION

Water intake is also an essential element that is often overlooked. Are you calculating how much water you drink in a day? Many clients I work with are barely getting in 4 cups (about 1 L) a day. That is not nearly enough to help support detoxification, optimize bowel movements and encourage weight loss.

Aim to drink at least half your body weight (in pounds) in ounces of water. For example, someone weighing 200 pounds (91 kg) would drink 100 ounces (2.8 L) of water daily. I also suggest adding in ½ teaspoon of high-quality sea salt to every quart (960 ml) of drinking water. Water alone will not hydrate the body, which is why electrolytes are just as important. Electrolytes are often lost through both physical and emotional stress, so it is important to hydrate with key electrolytes such as potassium, sodium and magnesium. Quality sea salt will provide these for you.

Our bodies are made up of over 70 percent water. Without proper hydration, we will very quickly impair normal bodily function. For health, body composition, athletic performance, detoxification, energy and vitality, it is extremely important that we drink adequate amounts of water.

Think about this: If we are made up of 70 percent water, and we consume high-quality water regularly, that's 70 percent of our health right there! However, tap water doesn't cut it. I recommend fresh springwater. Visit www .findaspring.com to locate a fresh spring near you.

MAIN BENEFITS OF OPTIMAL WATER INTAKE

1. Helps control cortisol levels. Cortisol is a stress hormone that can cause excessive weight gain and oxidative stress to the brain. High cortisol levels also impair your ability to build muscle.

2. Helps regulate body temperature. This is especially important during exercise. If you're dehydrated, you won't see the beautiful tone in your muscles.

3. Delivers nutrients and oxygen throughout the body.

4. Helps detoxify your kidneys and liver, especially from environmental pollution and the poisons we unknowingly eat.

5. Helps with the absorption of your vitamins and minerals.

6. Helps protect your body from injury by lubricating the joints.

7. Helps improve digestion. We need lots of fluids for our digestive system to function well.

8. Relieves constipation. Without water, we couldn't eliminate waste and other toxins in our bowels.

9. Fires up our metabolism. Cold water stimulates thermogenesis (i.e., burns calories!).

10. Prevents fatigue. If you're tired, drink a large glass of water. It will turn on those brain cells by allowing more oxygen to get to your brain.

It's also important to ditch plastic water bottles; they are full of toxins that can leach into your water. The worst part is, plastic is full of xenoestrogens—a "fake" estrogen that can mimic your natural estrogen hormone.

Xenoestrogens have been linked to many reproductive and hormonal cancers. This is scary stuff! Estrogen dominance comes with many symptoms, including weight gain, infertility, period pain, breast tenderness, headaches and water retention, just to name a few. Get yourself a glass water bottle. This is the safest option for your health, hormones and, of course, the planet.

Outside of bottle quality, water quality is of utmost importance. I personally like springwater, with reverse osmosis being a close second as long as it's remineralized. To me, it just makes sense to drink water that naturally flows through the earth, picks up good minerals from the soil and is intelligent enough to purify itself. Springwater is one of the only sources on this planet that has been untouched by pollution.

What about tap water? Personally, I don't recommend it. It's often loaded with fluoride and chlorine, chemicals that were added to our water in an effort to protect our health—so much for that!

Chlorine helps kill waterborne bacteria, but you don't want to be drinking it! It needs to be filtered out. Chlorine is a known hormone disruptor, particularly mimicking estrogen in our body. With breast tissue being so sensitive to estrogen and containing many estrogen receptors, this could pose a serious health risk for breast cancer.

As for fluoride, it has been deemed a toxic poison. Many countries have removed it from their drinking water because of this. In fact, fluoride in toothpaste damages the gums and disrupts collagen production. Imagine what it's doing to our teeth and health just by drinking it?

It's also important to note that tap water does not filter out medications. You could be drinking your neighbor's birth control pills or cholesterol-lowering drugs! These drugs get into the drinking water supply through several routes: some people flush unneeded medications down toilets and others pass the rest out in urine or feces. Some pharmaceuticals remain even after the wastewater treatments and cleansing done by water treatment plants.

If drinking plain ol' water bores you, then sista, there's nothing else I can say except to suck it up and start drinking. There are many ways to spruce up your water and make it more interesting, boosting the flavor without any added sugars and sweeteners.

A FEW OF MY FAVORITE WATER BLENDS

- Cucumber and lemon
- Frozen raspberries and mint
- Lime and pineapple
- Mint, lime and watermelon
- Orange, lemon and basil

Add one of these herbal combinations to your glass water bottle and *violà*! You've got a flavorful and delicious water to drink throughout the day.

DETOXIFICATION

We live in an age of information saturation. With so much misleading health information—often giving conflicting advice—even my most knowledgeable clients end up confused about what to eat.

My mission in life is to teach busy people how to make clean eating a way of life and how to regularly eliminate toxins, safely and effectively. Toxic overload can lead to fatigue, food allergies, weight gain, hormonal imbalance and a host of health issues.

Regularly detoxing allows you to enjoy:

- More energy
- Better moods
- Improved concentration
- Improved digestion and bowel elimination
- Reduced bloating and gas
- Fewer food allergies
- Weight loss or gain, as needed
- Hormonal balance
- Better skin
- Better sleep

So, let's harness that spring-cleaning energy, throw open the windows and get rid of the internal clutter—both physical and mental.

WHAT IS DETOXIFICATION?

Detoxification is about resting, cleansing and nourishing the body from the inside out. First you remove and eliminate toxins, then you feed your body with healthy nutrients. Detoxifying can help protect you from disease and renew your ability to maintain optimum health.

Detox has become such a buzzword, and clients often ask me why they should detox. I find that people often think they can run out to the nearest health food store, buy a 10-day detox kit and they will be fully detoxed in 10 days! Unfortunately, it doesn't work that way.

We detox *every single day*. So, as much as a detox kit may help, it's more important to think about the choices we make daily with our food and how we manage stress. We also need to pay attention to the toxin load we are exposed to in our cosmetics and household cleaning products—this is how we can *truly* assist our bodies and aid detoxification.

No matter how cleanly we eat, we live in a very toxic world. Before we even open our mouths to take a bite of food, we are exposed to industrial pollution in the air and toxins in our cleaning products and cosmetics. Not to mention the havoc wreaked on the body by stress. The question is not "Am I toxic?" but rather, "How toxic am I?"

Not that long ago we didn't have processed foods, mass agriculture or the levels of pollution we face today. Our bodies detox naturally, but they have not evolved fast enough to keep up with the increasing toxic load. When the body's natural detoxification systems reach their limit, we begin to experience symptoms of over-toxicity. This can lead to a host of health issues, such as:

- Fatigue
- Food allergies or intolerances
- Skin problems
- Weight gain or inability to gain weight
- Irritable bowel syndrome, constipation or irregular bowel movements
- Sluggish immune system
- Headaches and migraines
- Joint pain and inflammation
- Hormonal imbalances
- Depression, anxiety or constant mood swings
- Trouble sleeping
- Low sex drive
- Sugar cravings
- High blood pressure
- Increased acidity
- Osteoporosis
- Diabetes
- Heart disease
- Infertility
- Disrupted sleep patterns

DETOXIFYING FOODS

HERE ARE A FEW OF MY FAVORITE DETOX FOODS. ADD THESE TO YOUR RECIPES AND MAKE THEM A PART OF YOUR DIET FOR ADDED LIVER SUPPORT.

FOOD	BENEFITS
ARTICHOKE	GREAT FOR THE LIVER AND THE GALLBLADDER BECAUSE IT INCREASES BILE FLOW. IT IS ALSO A GREAT PREBIOTIC.
ASPARAGUS	CLEANSES THE KIDNEYS AND REDUCES WATER RETENTION. IT IS ALSO HIGH IN GLUTATHIONE AND FOLATE.
BEETS	A WONDERFUL BLOOD CLEANSER AND LOADED WITH ANTIOXIDANTS AND MINERALS.
DANDELION GREENS OR TEA	STIMULATES DIGESTIVE JUICES, HELPS DIGEST FATS AND SUPPORTS THE BODY'S NATURAL DETOXIFICATION PROCESSES. CAN ALSO BE ENJOYED AS A TEA.
FRESH HERBS	PARSLEY, CILANTRO AND BASIL ARE AMAZING CHELATORS. THEY HELP BIND TO HEAVY METALS AND FLUSH THEM FROM YOUR SYSTEM.
GARLIC	LOADED WITH ANTIBACTERIAL, ANTIVIRAL, ANTIFUNGAL AND ANTICANCER PROPERTIES. ONE OF NATURE'S BEST ANTIOXIDANTS.
LEAFY GREENS	KALE, SWISS CHARD, SPINACH, BOK CHOY, MUSTARD GREENS AND WATERCRESS ARE ALL RICH IN MAGNESIUM, WHICH IS AN IMPORTANT DETOXIFYING MINERAL.
NETTLE	RICH IN ANTIOXIDANTS, HIGH IN IRON AND GREAT FOR STRENGTHENING THE LIVER AND KIDNEYS. ALSO GREAT TO CONSUME IF YOU HAVE HEAVY PERIODS.
SEA VEGETABLES	DULSE, NORI, KELP, ARAME AND KOMBU ALL SUPPLY MINERALS AND IODINE TO HELP SUPPORT THE THYROID, IMMUNE SYSTEM AND LIVER DETOX PATHWAYS.
SUPERFOODS	CHLORELLA, SPIRULINA, CHLOROPHYLL AND WILD BLUE ALGAE ARE INCREDIBLY SUPPORTIVE FOR THE LIVER, GUT AND IMMUNE SYSTEM AND SUPPLY YOUR BODY WITH VITAL NUTRIENTS.

DETOXIFYING SPICES AND HERBS

SPICES AND HERBS ARE A GREAT WAY TO SUPPORT LIVER DETOXIFICATION,
PLUS THEY HELP BOOST FLAVOR IN YOUR MEALS WITHOUT USING SUGAR.
HERE ARE A FEW OF MY FAVORITES.

ANISE:
SOOTHES
THE DIGESTIVE TRACT

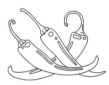

CAYENNE:
STIMULATES CIRCULATION,
BOOSTS THE IMMUNE SYSTEM

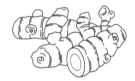

TURMERIC:
IS A POTENT ANTI-INFLAMMATORY
THAT NATURALLY
DETOXIFIES THE LIVER

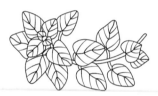

OREGANO:
CONTAINS ANTIBACTERIAL
PROPERTIES AND IS GREAT
FOR THE IMMUNE SYSTEM

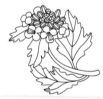

MUSTARD POWDER:
CONTAINS
ANTI-INFLAMMATORY
PROPERTIES

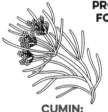

CUMIN:
RELIEVES GAS AND
SUPPORTS DIGESTION

CINNAMON:
REGULATES BLOOD SUGAR
AND AIDS DIGESTION

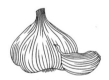

GARLIC POWDER:
REGULATES BLOOD
PRESSURE

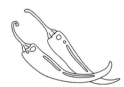

CHILI POWDER:
IS ANTI-INFLAMMATORY
AND SPEEDS
THE METABOLISM

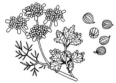

CORIANDER:
PROTECTS AGAINST
URINARY TRACT INFECTIONS
AND AIDS DIGESTION

If you suffer from any of the issues listed on page 70, it's time to hit your body's reset button by detoxing. Even if you aren't experiencing symptoms, it's recommended that everyone detox seasonally to give the body's detox organs a break.

THE ROLE OF THE LIVER IN DETOXIFICATION

Your liver is your main detoxifying organ. Bile is produced in the liver and stored in the gallbladder. A toxic and overburdened liver leads to impaired release of bile from the gallbladder; this affects the breakdown of fats and overall digestion. Bile is an important digestive fluid that helps in emulsifying fats. If you find you have digestive or abdominal pain, are vomiting or nauseated or experience fatty stools, this could mean you have a low-functioning gallbladder. Bile helps with bowel movements, and this is essential for eliminating excess estrogen. Thousands of women are dealing with estrogen dominance symptoms such as breast tenderness, bloating, headaches and migraines, water retention and weight gain.

FIVE ESSENTIAL ELEMENTS TO SUPPORT LIVER HEALTH

1. Ensure proper digestion and elimination.
2. Avoid environmental toxins/stressors.
3. Increase water and fiber intake.
4. Avoid excessive alcohol and refined sugar.
5. Ensure a healthy clean diet and appropriate supplementation.

Good health rests on the condition of our cells. Healthy cells require these four essentials: oxygen; healthy foods containing nutrients, minerals and plenty of antioxidants; adequate hydration; and well-functioning detoxification pathways.

What you eat is so important, and that's why the meals designed for you in this program are essential for your health and detoxification. By following this program, you will help release toxins, improve cellular energy and optimize your hormonal health.

THE CONNECTION BETWEEN THE LIVER AND ESTROGEN

Your liver is such an important detox organ, but beyond that it helps metabolize your hormones. It is *essential* in supporting overall hormonal health. Certain liver-detox enzymes help convert estrogen into its metabolites: 2-OHE1, 4-OHE1 and 16-OHE1.

Bear with me for a minute as I explain the importance of these different metabolites. First, 2-OHE1 is considered a "good estrogen," and it does not stimulate cell growth. It can help block the action of stronger, potentially carcinogenic estrogens. On the other hand, 4-OHE1 may directly damage DNA and cause mutations, which enhances cancer development. Also, 16-OHE1 has significant estrogenic activity, and studies show it may be associated with an increased risk of breast cancer. Studies show that higher levels of 16-OHE1 are associated with obesity, hypothyroidism, pesticide toxicity (organochlorines), too much omega-6 fatty acids and inflammatory cytokines.

Basically, we want to get your estrogen to the favorable 2-OHE1 metabolite. This happens by eating your veggies—more specifically, cruciferous vegetables. Listen, I don't mean to scare you and bring up the big C word (cancer). But if you're avoiding your veggies like the plague and complaining about how you just don't like broccoli, it is time to suck it up and get creative with your food. Follow the recipes in this program—which will help you love your veggies—and protect your body, hormones, breasts and ovaries by eating your vegetables.

There are many vegetables that resonate with the liver's energy: think broccoli, dandelion, cauliflower and scallions. Warming herbs and spices such as garlic, ginger and cinnamon are beneficial, as are the sour tastes of lemons and limes. Vinegar-based or pickled foods are also used to support liver function.

LIVER DETOXIFICATION

Your liver goes through two detoxification phases in order to eliminate wastes and toxins. In phase 1, the liver works to neutralize chemicals and wastes, making them "weak" or water-soluble so they can be effectively eliminated in phase 2.

In phase 2, these toxins become altered by various chemicals, which further neutralizes them or eliminates them through the gut. It's important that we provide the right nutrients and foods to help the liver during these two phases. The charts on pages 71–72 show my favorite foods, herbs and spices for supporting detoxification.

SUPPORT PHASE 1 DETOXIFICATION

- Eat cruciferous vegetables, such as broccoli, cauliflower, cabbage and Brussels sprouts.

- Include citrus fruits, such as lemons and limes.

- Load up on vitamin C–rich foods, such as strawberries, papaya, peppers and kale.

- Include vitamin E–rich foods, such as avocados, sunflower seeds and almonds.

- Include anti-inflammatory turmeric or the supplement curcumin in your diet.

- Supplement with vitamin C and a vitamin B complex.

SUPPORT PHASE 2 DETOXIFICATION

- Cruciferous vegetables are also important here. Broccoli, cauliflower, Brussels sprouts and cabbage are great options.

- Include pasture-raised organic eggs.

- Eat sulfur-containing foods, such as garlic, onions, leeks and shallots.

- Be sure to hydrate with 3 liters (12.5 cups) of water daily.

- Include glutathione-rich foods, such as asparagus, walnuts and avocados.

- Be sure to eat adequate amounts of protein.

- Supplement with vitamin C and a vitamin B complex.

It should go without saying that to effectively support your liver and detox pathways, alcohol, coffee, sugar and nicotine should be eliminated or dramatically reduced.

GLUTATHIONE: AN ANTIOXIDANT POWERHOUSE

Glutathione is a powerful antioxidant produced by the liver. During phase 1 and phase 2 of detoxification, glutathione will step in and help to neutralize any free radical damage and assist in the detoxification process. Food sources of glutathione include walnuts, asparagus and avocados. Be sure to include them in your diet weekly for extra liver support.

I also highly recommend supplementing with liposomal glutathione, which is especially important for those dealing with autoimmune Hashimoto's or thyroid issues in general. You can also find this in topical form and apply it directly over your thyroid to help protect it against free radicals and lower autoimmune antibodies. As for internally, I highly recommend the liposomal form, as it is more easily assimilated. I use the one from Designs for Health. For more details about this product, go to my shop page at shop.holisticwellness.ca.

BROCCOPROTECT

I am a huge fan of the supplement BroccoProtect from Designs for Health. You'd have to consume over 1 pound (450 g) of broccoli or nearly ¼ pound (113 g) of broccoli sprouts to get the same amount of sulforaphane in 1 capsule. Brocco-Protect helps to support phase 2 detoxification of the liver, helps to detox out excess estrogens and has many anticancer protective properties. Keep in mind, nothing will ever replace eating fruits and vegetables, but supplements can absolutely be helpful in addition to a whole foods diet.

LIVER SUPPORT AND DETOX BRANDS AND SUPPLEMENTS I LOVE

- N-Acetyl Cysteine by Designs for Health or Advanced Orthomolecular Research
- SC Liver Formula by Alpha Science Laboratories
- Cleanse Smart by Renew Life
- Turmeric by Integrative Therapeutics
- HepatoDR by St. Francis Herb Farm
- Milk Thistle tincture by St. Francis Herb Farm
- Detox Kit by Pascoe
- B-Supreme by Designs for Health
- B Complex by Advanced Orthomolecular Research
- BroccoProtect by Designs for Health
- Liposomal Vitamin C by Designs for Health
- Liposomal Glutathione by Designs for Health
- Vitamin C from NOW foods, Advanced Orthomolecular Research or Sisu
- Oceans Alive by Activation Products

LOVING YOUR LIVER DAILY

By now you've seen just how important the liver is in maintaining optimal hormonal health. Here are my top suggestions for loving your liver and reducing its workload.

1. Eliminate the toxic load of what you ingest through food and drink. Try to eat organic when possible. Cut out alcohol during this detox and/or keep alcohol consumption moderate going forward. Alcohol slows down the detoxification process and impairs the health of the liver.

2. Reduce toxins in your home by choosing natural beauty products and cleaning products when possible.

3. Consume lemon water or apple cider vinegar upon waking. Or whip up my antiaging elixir—1 cup (240 ml) warm water, a squeeze of lemon juice, ½ tablespoon (8 ml) of apple cider vinegar (optional) and ½ scoop of collagen powder.

4. Stay hydrated by drinking half your body weight in ounces of water daily. For a boost in cellular regeneration and liver support, add 1 teaspoon of chlorophyll, spirulina or any greens powder to 10 ounces (284 ml) of water. Consume up to three times a day during this program if you like. You can find these at your local health food store or try out PaleoGreens, one of my favorites, at www.shop.holisticwellness.ca. I advise against spirulina or chlorella if you have an autoimmune condition, as they can be immune stimulating.

5. Support a healthy colon by drinking flax tea—add 1 tablespoon (10 g) of ground flaxseeds to 1 cup (240 ml) of water. Or add extra fiber, such as chia or flaxseeds, to meals or smoothies. Fiber is vital for removing toxic wastes from the colon. Keep in mind, the toxins your liver breaks down are then sent to the colon for elimination. Optimizing bowel movements and gut health is essential for detoxification.

6. Eat foods that naturally cleanse the liver, such as apples, lemons, limes, asparagus, broccoli, radishes, cucumbers, spinach, watercress, parsley, cilantro and bitter greens.

7. Close the kitchen two to three hours before bedtime. Sleep is when the liver begins to clean the body of wastes. If you find you are hungry before bed, drink 8 ounces (240 ml) of water with a pinch of sea salt.

SIMPLE AT-HOME DETOX PROTOCOLS

As you follow along with the 30-Day Hormone Solution meal plan, I suggest you include these at-home detox protocols daily or a couple of times throughout the week. This will take your detox to a whole new level by helping your body to release toxins, supporting your parasympathetic nervous system, improving your gut health and improving your sleep—all things essential for optimizing your hormonal health.

AYURVEDIC ABHYANGA MASSAGE

Abhyanga is known as the Ayurvedic oil massage. It is an integral part in Ayurvedic medicine. This simple, luxurious massage is wonderful for reducing stress hormones, improving sleep and supporting overall health. Here are some of the benefits traditionally associated with regular abhyanga massage:

- Increases circulation, especially to nerve endings
- Moves the lymph, aiding in detoxification
- Tones the muscles
- Calms the nerves
- Lubricates the joints
- Increases mental alertness
- Softens skin
- Improves deep sleep at night

Administering the abhyanga massage can help purify the skin, which is the largest organ in the body. This purification assists the skin in performing its diverse functions efficiently and allowing toxins to be released from the body. Think of it like oiling the engine of your car—if you do it regularly, your engine will be in peak condition, and give you years and years of trouble-free performance.

Abhyanga is traditionally performed in the morning upon waking, or in the evening before bed, before your bath or shower, to facilitate the release of toxins that may have accumulated during the previous night or over the course of the day. Sesame oil or jojoba oil is traditionally used for this massage, so when purchasing oils, be sure to look for cold-pressed, chemical-free organic sesame or jojoba oil. Both oils contain antioxidants that are wonderful for protecting the skin against free radical damage.

To begin your massage, simply heat your bottle of oil under running hot water. Remove it from the heat once the desired temperature is reached, aiming for a temperature that isn't too hot and is comfortable on your body without causing any burn.

Place oil into the palm of your hands and apply it lightly to your entire body, starting with your face and working your way down to your toes. Massage the oil into your skin in circular motions and use long strokes on your limbs. Always massage toward the direction of your heart. As an option, you can start from the crown of your head, applying oil to your hair and massaging your scalp.

Apply light pressure on sensitive areas, such as the abdomen or the heart. Use more oil and spend more time where your nerve endings are concentrated, such as the soles of the feet, palms of the hands and along the base of the fingernails.

After you're done, relax for 10 to 15 minutes, letting the oil and the massage work its magic. The longer the oil is on, the deeper it penetrates into your skin. During this time, you can read something relaxing or uplifting, or rest and lie on a towel on your bed. I prefer to perform this massage at night and follow it up with a warm bath or shower. Once in the shower, I wash only my dirty parts (aka—armpits and lady parts), which are the most important, with soap. Keep in mind that your microbiome doesn't just live in your gut, but also on your skin. Constant washing and cleaning of the skin can deplete our delicate microbiome, which is essential in supporting our immune defenses.

INFRARED SAUNA

Infrared is truly the best detoxification treat you can give yourself. In a regular sauna the heat penetrates your surface skin. The heat is really only warming up the air around you, whereas in an infrared sauna, the heat penetrates deep into your subcutaneous fat cells. Yup ... ya heard right—I said fat cells! You see, toxins get stored in our fat cells. Our fat cells become a safe haven for heavy metals and chemicals, such as mercury, cadmium and lead; pesticides; herbicides and BPA.

Infrared is one of the best ways to help eliminate these toxins. Our skin has the ability to access these fat stores through sweating. Essentially, when you're sitting in a hot sauna, your core body temperature begins to rise. In turn, your blood vessels dilate, enhancing blood flow. Once the brain is signaled, your sweat glands are stimulated to cool your body down. Toxins in your body tissues are then mobilized and eliminated via sweat.

Regular exposure to infrared can help trigger heat shock proteins (HSPs), which can prevent cellular damage by directly scavenging free radicals and helping to maintain glutathione levels. What is also interesting is that exposure to heat has been shown to increase life span (by up to 15 percent) in flies and worms, a benefit that is attributed to HSPs. One particular HSP (the HSP70 gene) has also been associated with increased longevity, which suggests there may be antiaging benefits to regular heat stress.

BENEFITS OF USING AN INFRARED SAUNA

- Improves liver detoxification
- Eliminates toxins and heavy metals through sweat
- Improves skin health
- Lowers blood pressure
- Reduces stress
- Accelerates healing
- Improves circulation
- Eases muscle aches and pains

Note: If you are dealing with cancer, it's important to undergo a medically supervised treatment plan.

Find a local spa in your area that has an infrared sauna where you can pay by the session, or consider purchasing one for your home. When purchasing a sauna, be sure find one that is made with the most natural materials. Often, saunas can be made with harmful formaldehyde, toxic glue, chemical fire retardants, plastic or fiberglass heaters. The last thing you want is to be detoxing in a sauna full of chemicals.

Aim for three or four sauna sessions a week if you can, or daily if you have one at home. Start with 15-minute sessions, working your way up to 30 minutes. After sauna use, be sure to replenish electrolytes with either water, ½ teaspoon of sea salt and a scoop of quality greens powder, the Post-Workout Recovery Shake (page 154) or the Ginger Turmeric Lemonade (page 157; just be sure to add some sea salt to the lemonade). Your electrolytes are important for balancing internal fluid levels, as well as regulating muscle and nerve activity.

DRY SKIN BRUSHING

Our skin is our largest organ and responsible for one-fourth of our body's daily detoxification, which is huge. Dry skin brushing can help assist your body with proper toxin elimination and cleanse your lymphatic system of toxins that accumulate in your lymph glands. It also aids in increasing circulation, helps open pores and truly invigorates your skin. Every day we are exposed to toxins, both from food and the environment. If we cannot properly eliminate these toxins, our skin will be one of the many organs that suffers. Cell renewal will take longer, wrinkles become more apparent; acne, eczema or psoriasis can worsen; and our everyday glow will start to fade.

It's important to use a brush made with natural bristles, not synthetic, so it won't scratch the surface of your skin. A long handle would be great as well to reach inaccessible areas of your back.

BENEFITS OF REGULAR DRY SKIN BRUSHING

- Rids your body of metabolic wastes
- Encourages cell regeneration
- Increases blood flow
- Lessens the appearance of cellulite
- Improves muscle tone
- Eliminates dead skin cells
- Improves lymphatic congestion, which in turn will support estrogen detox
- Decreases symptoms such as breast tenderness around your cycle

HOW TO DRY BRUSH

- Always dry brush before getting into the shower. Brushing on wet skin will not have the same effects on cell regeneration.
- Begin with long sweeping strokes, starting from the soles of your feet. Work upward toward your legs and thighs.
- From your hands, work up toward your elbows and toward your shoulders. Brush across your stomach and buttocks.
- Try to brush upward from your lower back to your neck.
- Strokes should always be toward the heart.
- Brush several times in each area.

Try to dry brush first thing in the morning. Afterward, try alternating between hot and cold water in the shower to further stimulate circulation and bring blood to the surface of your skin. Always begin with hot and end with cold. Alternating hot and cold showers is just another therapeutic way to invigorate your skin, ease muscle soreness and enhance overall health and energy.

To further support detoxification and gut health, perform a lymphatic drainage massage to the outside and inside of your thighs after dry skin brushing. Rubbing the outside of your thighs vigorously helps with drainage from the large intestine, while the inside of your thighs will stimulate drainage of the small intestine.

EPSOM SALT BATHS

A simple way to unwind in the evening and detox your body is with Epsom salt baths. Simply fill your tub with warm to hot water, and add 2 cups (300 g) of Epsom salts. Feel free to add essential oils, such as lavender, or even a few tablespoons of jojoba oil to help soften your skin while soaking. Epsom salt is not really a salt but rather a compound of magnesium and sulfate. These are easily absorbed through the skin, which makes an Epsom salt bath a great way to replenish your body of the much-needed magnesium. Including an Epsom salt bath a few times a week is wonderful for supporting your parasympathetic nervous system, easing stress, assisting with sleep and reducing inflammation and pain.

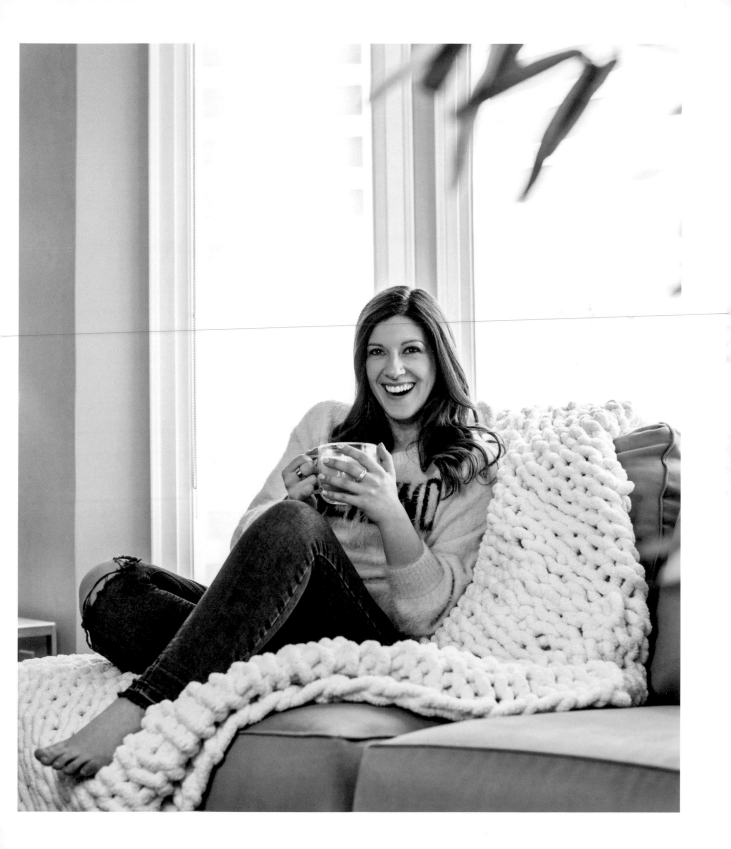

CASTOR OIL PACKS

I remember studying women's health and endocrine disorders in school more than ten years ago, and I learned how castor oil can be used to help shrink cysts and fibroids. I will never forget that day, as it led me to a regular routine of using castor oil packs for my hormones and liver health. In fact, castor oil can help dissolve scar tissue, making it a great oil to keep on hand if you are an athlete, train regularly or are recovering from a surgery.

Castor oil packs for liver detox: If you've never heard of castor oil packs, they are traditionally used to help detox the liver and assist with gallbladder disorders. They are wonderful for digestive and gastrointestinal issues such as IBS, constipation, cramping or bloating. They are also great for painful PMS cramps, uterine fibroids, endometriosis and nonmalignant ovarian cysts. I often use castor oil packs before bed and before I know it, I'm sound asleep. Not only does the oil have an amazing affinity to help cleanse and "move" toxins out through your system, but it's also very calming.

Take a piece of flannel, approximately the size of your hand, and saturate it with a high-quality, cold-pressed castor oil. You can infuse your castor oil with dried lavender or add a few drops of lavender essential oil for an extra calming effect. Lay the flannel on top of your liver—located on the right side of your body, just under your ribs. Place a hot water bottle on top.

Note: Do not use an electric heating pad. Lie down, close your eyes and breathe deeply. The oil actually penetrates deep through the layers of your skin to help cleanse and remove toxins from your liver. The healing components of the oil, known as ricinoleic acid, penetrate directly into your tissues.

You can use warm water and soap to wash the oil off, or if you aren't bothered by the oil, you can leave it on your skin all night and go to bed. It can sometimes stain your clothes or sheets, so be conscious of this if you don't want to make a mess. Truthfully, I've never had an issue with this. You can reuse your piece of flannel over and over again. Store it in a ziplock bag or container, and add a few extra drops of oil each time you reuse it. Replace the flannel once it starts to change color.

From boobs to pubes—castor oil for cysts and fibroids: That's right, you heard me say it—from boobs to pubes. This is my favorite way to use castor oil.

With this method, I would advise that you mix castor oil with another lighter oil, such as olive oil. A mixture of 50 percent castor oil with 50 percent olive oil is a good blend. Keep in mind that a little bit of castor oil goes a long way. Once you've blended your oils together, apply oil "from boobs to pubes," massaging all over your breasts, stomach, liver and all the way down over your ovaries and to your pubic bone.

Because castor oil encourages lymphatic drainage, it can help to shrink cysts and fibroids. It works by increasing the efficiency of circulation to your pelvis. Good circulation is required for supportive nutrients to be delivered to your cells, and for waste products and inflammatory chemicals to be removed.

Due to the oil increasing circulation, you may want to avoid using the oil during your period if you tend to have a heavier flow. Typically, the oil can help to decrease menstrual cramping and breast tenderness, so apply it onto your body the week prior to your period. Otherwise, be sure to monitor your flow if you do decide to use the oil throughout your period. As noted above, I like to leave the oil on all night and go to bed. I find I sleep more soundly, and it helps me to relax. However, you can leave it on your skin for at least 30 minutes, then gently wash it off.

REAL TALK

If you are in an adrenally depleted state, plus are dealing with the onset of an autoimmune condition, overexercising, HIIT (high-intensity interval training) or cardio are not ideal. I was stuck in the mentality that if I wasn't pushing my body hard enough or sweating enough, I wasn't making any physical changes, but unfortunately, that type or exercise just left me completely depleted.

You must take time to heal your body first and slow down. In fact, for the first two weeks of your 30-day reset, I suggest you only include parasympathetic exercise, such as yoga or walking, before increasing the intensity of your workouts. For me, it took nearly eight months before I could get back to heavy lifting and more regular exercise. I spent those first eight months doing light yoga, walking and Pilates-style classes, but more than anything, I focused on my sleep. It was a combination of sleep, daily strategic supplementation and supporting my gut health that ultimately gave me my energy back. Now I work out three to four days a week, focusing primarily on lifting weights with some lighter forms of HIIT. And more than anything, I pay attention to how I feel. Some days I wake up and feel like going for a walk. Other days I have the energy to weight train or include some hill sprints or run the stairs.

Luckily, we now live closer to parks, hiking and biking trails and a gorgeous lake where we go kayaking in the summer and spend a lot of time outside engaging in summer activities. What is key for me though, and made a huge impact with my exercise, was taking longer breaks in between sets, versus pushing myself to go faster and harder. Slowing down my exercise made all the difference. I get to reap the benefits of weight training while keeping my energy levels stable. If you find yourself exhausted after a cardio-type class or working out in general, you most likely need to work on healing your adrenals and managing your stress first.

EXERCISE

We can't talk about detoxification without speaking about exercise, which just so happens to be one of the best ways to detox your body and sweat out those toxins. You've probably heard the saying before, "You can't out-exercise a bad diet." Over the years, I've coached many women who struggled to give up sugar or their daily glass of wine and change their diet. Yet, they work out five to seven days a week with little to no results. If you want to optimize your results in the gym, it starts in your kitchen.

As a child, I was incredibly active. In fact, I am grateful that I grew up in an era without cell phones and social media. I spent every day outside in the garden, in the backyard, riding my bike around my neighborhood and getting dirty in the playground. Exercise was a part of my daily life and continued well into my teens, twenties and beyond. I started lifting weights and going to the gym at sixteen years old, and then I taught kickboxing, Pilates and yoga classes and I absolutely loved lifting heavy weights.

WEIGHT TRAINING CIRCUIT

DO AS MANY ROUNDS AS POSSIBLE IN 30 MINUTES,
RESTING AS NEEDED.

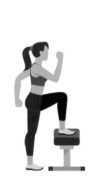
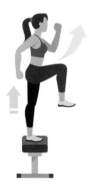
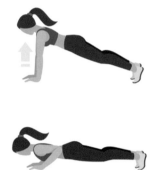
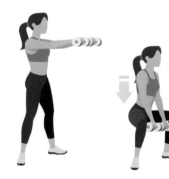

10 X STEP UPS HOLDING A DUMBBELL IN EACH HAND
EXERCISE CAN BE PERFORMED WITH OR WITHOUT DUMBBELLS

10 X PUSHUPS

10 X DUMBBELL SWINGS (OR DUMBBELL DEADLIFTS AS A SUBSTITUTE)

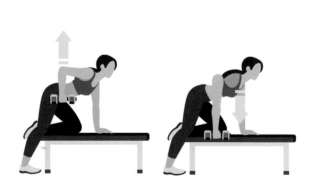
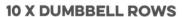
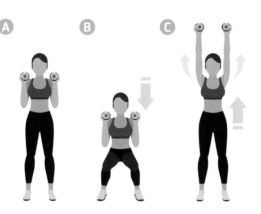

10 X DUMBBELL ROWS

10 X DUMBBELL SQUAT TO PRESS

However, in 2017, when my autoimmune Hashimoto's symptoms were at their worst, I had a hard time lifting and gripping weights, and a typical HIIT class left me exhausted. I would literally come home after a workout class and fall asleep on the couch!

Exercise does not mean you need to get a gym membership. It's about moving your body. I have a client who loathes weight training and cardio classes, but loves all kinds of sports. She's active with her family throughout the entire year—snowboarding and skiing in the winter, and swimming and playing beach volleyball in the summer. This is her exercise, and she's inspired and excited to do it. Weight-bearing exercise is essential for women's health. If you don't engage in regular activity, I highly suggest picking up some weights; they will not only help to tone your muscles, but support bone density, which declines as we age.

Included on the previous page is a full-body workout circuit that I like to perform two days out of the week. It targets all major muscle groups and is also great when you are crunched for time. After your first two weeks on your reset, include this circuit two times a week—along with one or two yoga classes or walking and hiking throughout the week.

EMOTIONAL DETOX

Allowing emotional toxins to arise and release is just as important as the physical side of the detox. If you find emotions coming up, give yourself the space to sit with them. Journal, take a bath, go for a walk or talk to a trusted friend.

It's important to sit with uncomfortable emotions and not push them aside. I know it can be easy to disregard feelings of hurt, anger or fear. But sitting with these and understanding why they are showing up will allow you to work through them with greater emotional intelligence and awareness in the future.

Understanding your fears means you can better handle them when they do show up; this allows you to go from dealing with your fears in hours, to minutes to seconds. As you make your way through the reset, I encourage you to build up your compassion muscle. Think about how you would treat a hurt animal or a crying child. Probably with gentle kindness and love. And this is exactly the kind of treatment you need to give to yourself.

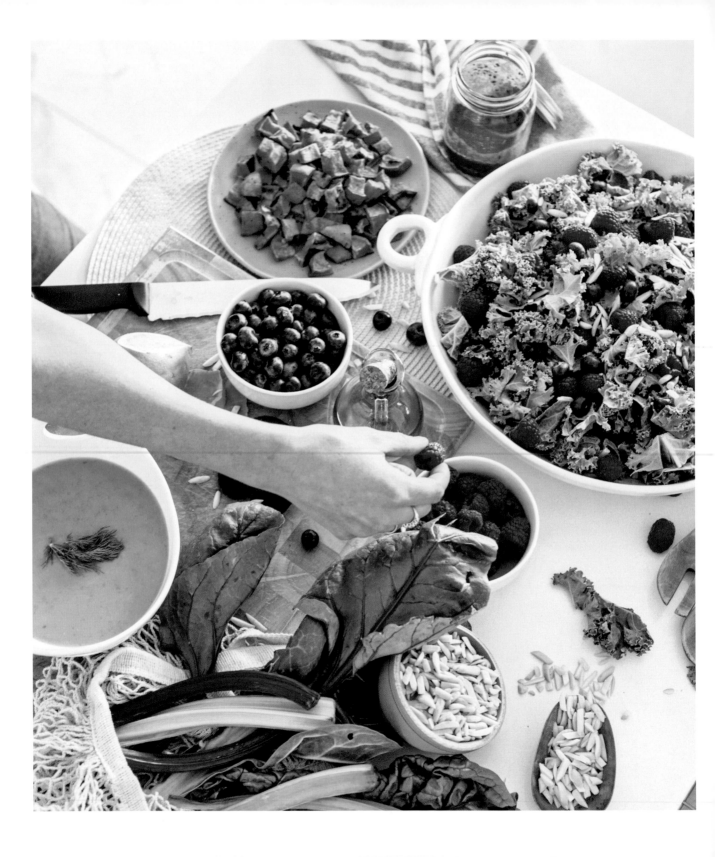

CHAPTER 8:

GUT HEALTH:

SIMPLE STEPS FOR OPTIMIZING YOUR MICROBIOME

Your gut is not just about your waistline or belly; it's the gateway to the health of your brain and immune system. Some two thousand years ago Hippocrates, an ancient Greek physician, said, "All disease begins in the gut." It seems now more than ever that we should start listening to this and look at where many of our health issues stem from: the gut. I believe that the future of medicine will focus primarily on restoring the integrity of the gut barrier, and rightfully so.

THE IMPORTANCE OF GUT HEALTH

Seventy million people suffer from digestive issues. In addition to that, fifteen million people suffer from food allergies of some form, and most aren't even aware of them.

My gut health has taken quite the hit over the years. I mentioned in previous chapters that I was a C-section baby, meaning I did not pass through the birth canal and pick up all that good bacteria to help inoculate my microbiome. I was also fed formula, put on many over-the-counter cold and flu meds as a kid, went on the birth control pill for seven years and caught a parasite on vacation in my mid-twenties that took a toll on my digestion and gut health. These things might seem fairly harmless, and growing up I had no idea nor did my parents about the impact they could have on my health.

The reality of the matter is, your gut health starts the moment you are born. And any medication use, toxin exposure, NSAIDs (e.g., ibuprofen) and stress, combined with a high-sugar diet, can all impact the integrity of your gut barrier.

WHAT CONTRIBUTES TO AN UNHEALTHY GUT

Gut health can be adversely impacted by the following:

- Antibiotics and other medications, such as birth control and NSAIDs
- Diets high in refined carbohydrates, sugar and processed foods
- Diets low in fermentable fibers
- Dietary toxins, such as wheat and gluten
- Industrial seed oils, such as soy, corn and other vegetable oils
- Chronic stress
- Chronic infections

Most of us think only of poop when we think of our gut. But gut health goes beyond just a daily bowel movement. Your gut bacteria assist in the breakdown of food and promote normal gastrointestinal function. Healthy gut flora (bacteria) impacts your vitality, immunity and hormones; protects you from food allergies and intolerances; and is essential for cognition, memory and brain health, as well as regulating metabolism.

There are two important areas to look at when we speak about gut health: your gut barrier, and your microbiota or "gut flora." Your gut *literally* impacts everything in the body and is deeply connected to all areas of your health. When your gut barrier is weakened, known as leaky gut, instead of excreting toxins, pathogens, food particles, drugs and infections through your bowels (poop), these substances get absorbed into your bloodstream. Instead of releasing these toxins, we end up retoxing our bodies by reabsorbing these things back into our bloodstream.

THE GUT BARRIER

Your gut barrier is like the gatekeeper that decides what gets in and what stays out. Think about it for a minute . . . anything that goes in the mouth and isn't digested will pass right out the other end. Your gut barrier protects your body from allowing foreign substances to enter. However, when the barrier becomes leaky or permeable, molecules escape into your bloodstream. Because these molecules do not belong in your bloodstream, your body mounts an immune response and attacks them. Studies show that these attacks play a role in the development of autoimmune disease, such as Hashimoto's and type 1 diabetes among others.

You don't have to have gut symptoms to have a leaky gut. This is crucial to understand. Many of the women I work with in my private practice look at me like I have three heads when I tell them we need to address their gut health. They respond with, "But I'm not bloated or gassy." Leaky gut can manifest as skin problems such as eczema, psoriasis, joint pain, autoimmunity, depression, mental illness and autism spectrum disorder. If you are dealing with any of these issues, without any real change in your symptoms, have you started on a gut-healing protocol? If not, now is the time to start. Leaky gut is often the root cause of many diseases, and unfortunately, conventional medical doctors have scoffed at the idea that a leaky gut can contribute to disease.

Many autoimmune diseases, such as celiac, type 2 diabetes, multiple sclerosis and rheumatoid arthritis, are characterized by abnormally high levels of zonulin, a protein that increases intestinal permeability and thereby leaky gut. One of the main reasons we want to avoid consuming wheat and other gluten products and grains is that they contain a protein called gliadin, which has been shown to increase zonulin production and is directly related to leaky gut. Have you ditched the gluten yet? Now is the time to start!

GUT FLORA

Basically, we are one big walking bug! Our gut is home to approximately 100 trillion microorganisms and contains ten times more bacteria than all the human cells in the entire body. Antibiotics are particularly harmful to your gut flora, causing a shift in their composition. This diversity of flora is not recovered after antibiotic use unless probiotics are incorporated as part of a gut-healing protocol. According to one study, infants that aren't breast-fed and are born to mothers with bad gut flora are more likely to develop unhealthy gut bacteria. These early differences in gut flora may predict overweight, diabetes, eczema, psoriasis, depression and other health problems in the future.

If you have bad gut flora, there is a good chance you also have leaky gut—and vice versa. If both your gut flora and your gut barrier are impaired, you will have inflammation, period. You may not feel it at first, but internally there is inflammation going on. And, at some point, if your gut health is left untreated, this will lead to disease and symptoms down the road. Thus, it is essential to rebuild your gut flora and restore intestinal permeability to adequately address these conditions.

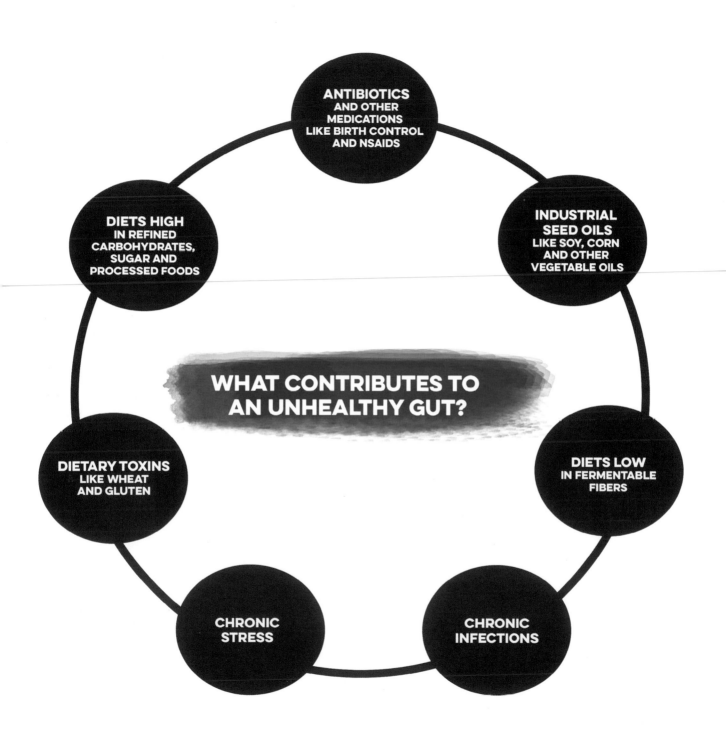

WHAT CONTRIBUTES TO
AN UNHEALTHY GUT?

ANTIBIOTICS
AND OTHER
MEDICATIONS
LIKE BIRTH CONTROL
AND NSAIDS

INDUSTRIAL
SEED OILS
LIKE SOY, CORN
AND OTHER
VEGETABLE OILS

DIETS HIGH
IN REFINED
CARBOHYDRATES,
SUGAR AND
PROCESSED FOODS

DIETS LOW
IN FERMENTABLE
FIBERS

DIETARY TOXINS
LIKE WHEAT
AND GLUTEN

CHRONIC
STRESS

CHRONIC
INFECTIONS

HOW LEAKY GUT PROGRESSES

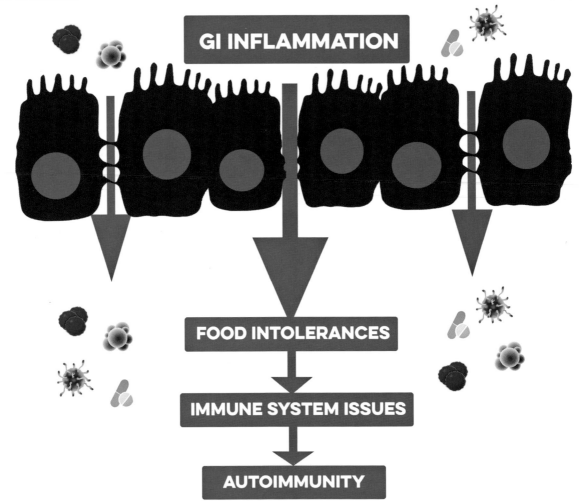

UNDIGESTED FOOD PARTICLES

TOXINS

STRESS

MEDICATION

PATHOGENS

ORGAN MALFUNCTION

GI INFLAMMATION

FOOD INTOLERANCES

IMMUNE SYSTEM ISSUES

AUTOIMMUNITY

STEPS TO HEALING YOUR GUT

1. Remove all food toxins, food intolerances and any potential food triggers. Wheat, gluten, dairy, soy, corn and eggs are often culprits, along with genetically modified organisms (GMOs), herbicides, insecticides and pesticides.

2. Eat plenty of fermentable fibers, such as sweet potatoes, yams, yucca and plantains.

3. Include fermented foods, such as sauerkraut, kimchi, kefir and raw dairy (if tolerated), and include a high-quality probiotic.

4. Consume 1 cup (240 ml) of bone broth daily to help heal the lining of the gut.

5. Test for intestinal pathogens (e.g. parasites, fungi, viruses, etc.), and treat them with strategic protocols.

6. Limit your alcohol and sugar intake.

7. Manage your stress levels.

8. Optimize your digestion by including digestive enzymes with your meals (I like NOW brand, Designs for Health or Enzymedica).

9. Consider taking ½ to 1 tablespoon (8 to 15 ml) of apple cider vinegar mixed with warm water daily to help with any acid reflux issues, or try supplementing with deglycyrrhizinated licorice (DGL).

Address nutrient deficiencies. If your diet is low in B_{12}, iron, vitamin C, selenium, zinc and magnesium *and* you have low stomach acid, your enzyme production will be impaired.

PROBIOTICS

Here's what you need to look for in a probiotic:

- Live active cultures
- No sugar added (typically used with cheaper brands)
- Enterically coated for serious digestive issues
- A combination of different strains, including *L. acidophilus* and *L. bifidus* bacteria
- At least 10 billion cultures or more if you need intensive gut healing
- Non-GMO certified

GUT-HEALING SUPPLEMENTS I LOVE

- GI Revive by Designs for Health
- Digestive Enzymes by NOW, Designs for Health or Enzymedica
- Probiotics by Design for Health, Mega-SporeBiotic, Renew Life or Genuine Health
- Aloe Vera juice or gel by Land Art
- LGS Gut Therapy Healing Fibre by Nu Life Therapeutics
- L-Glutamine by Advanced Orthomolecular Research
- Omega-3 fish oil by NutraSea or Designs for Health

Healing your gut takes time and patience, as with most things. It can also be confusing and complicated at times, especially if there are underlying infections going on that can be found only through testing. Working with a practitioner who can design a strategic gut-healing protocol will help you achieve faster results. Be sure to set realistic expectations when it comes to healing, and never give up on your journey to achieving the health and vitality you desire.

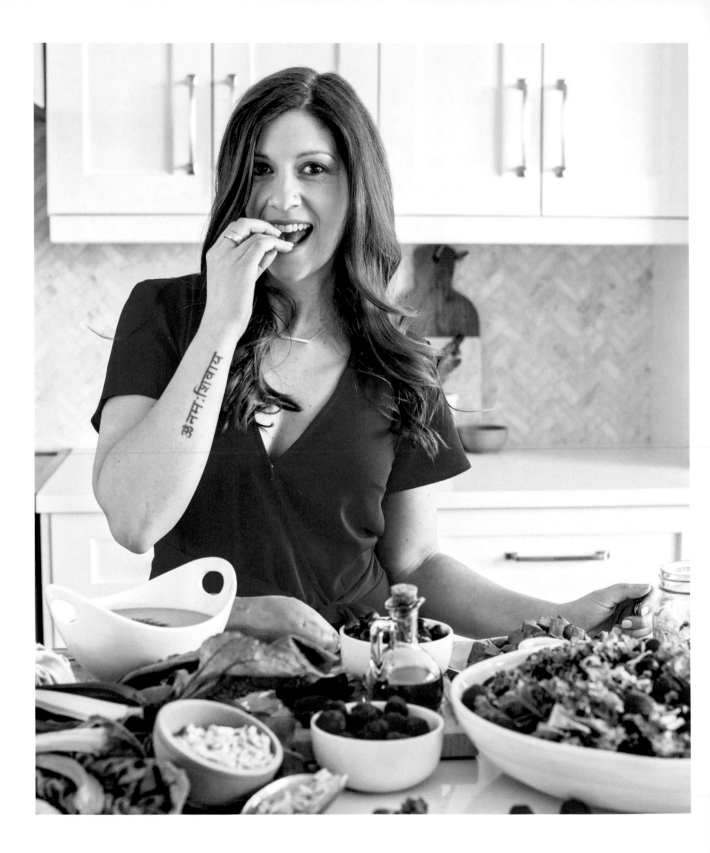

CHAPTER 9:

YOUR HORMONE SOLUTION RULES AND 30-DAY MEAL PLAN

When it comes to following the 30-Day Hormone Solution, there are important rules to follow in order to achieve optimal success. We've already discussed a few of these rules in previous chapters, but below you will find a complete list. Please take the time to read through each rule and implement them as best as you can.

Something that is important to note is that it's *okay to be hungry!* There's a good chance you won't feel hungry on this reset. But, if you're used to snacking and grazing, and now you are focusing on eating only three meals, you might find you're hungry for the first few days as your blood sugar balances out.

We are so used to the feeling of fullness that we don't even know what it means to be empty. Hunger pains are okay. Feeling empty is okay. Nothing bad is going to happen to you. A huge part of this program is about helping you balance out your blood sugar so you don't have to feel chained to food all the time. Take a deep breath when the hunger sets in, be sure to drink lots of water and you'll be just fine.

THE TEN HORMONE SOLUTION RULES

Reset Rule #1—No snacking. Eat only three meals a day, spacing your meals out roughly 4 to 6 hours apart. Gut Gummies (page 204), treats or elixirs should be included *as part of your meal and not a snack, if you decide to include them.*

Reset Rule #2—Hydrate. Aim to drink 3 liters (12.5 cups) of water a day. Outside of water, you can enjoy pure herbal, non-caffeinated teas *between* your meals.

Reset Rule #3—No alcohol, fruit juice, green juice, fresh-pressed juice or artificially sweetened juices/beverages are allowed during your reset.

Reset Rule #4—Limit yourself to one black coffee daily or enjoy the Coconut Collagen Coffee recipe on page 162. Enjoy your coffee *as part of* your meal. Avoid consuming it in between meals so as not to raise cortisol and insulin levels.

Note: Not all coffee is bad. Quality is key here. More importantly, what are you putting in your coffee? If your daily cup of java is a double-double, then it's time for a change. Opt for stevia or monk fruit as your sweetener, and try out nondairy nut milks, such as almond, cashew or coconut.

Reset Rule #5—Limit your intake of fruit to no more than three servings a day. Fruit can be enjoyed *as part of* your meals.

Reset Rule #6—No eating after 9 p.m. Aim to get in all of your meals before this time. However, our schedules can get the best of us, so I would rather you eat a late meal than no meal at all if you happen to get home after 9 p.m.

Reset Rule #7—Start your reset with the three-day liquid cleanse. All the recipes and information are laid out for you in your meal plan on pages 93–97.

Reset Rule #8—Include variety. You'll notice that your meal plan contains a different protein at each meal, along with veggies, fats and/or a starchy carb. Including a different protein at each meal ensures you are providing your body with an array of amino acids.

Reset Rule #9—Include a fourteen-hour intermittent fast at least two to three days out of the week. Outside of the fourteen hours, aim for twelve hours daily at the very least. You can work your way up to a sixteen-hour fast if you feel confident and comfortable doing so. This would mean fasting from dinner to breakfast for sixteen hours, then eating within an eight-hour window. In this case, it might make more sense to include only two meals a day versus three.

Reset Rule #10—Include daily light movement for the first two weeks of your program. This can be in the form of a daily walk or a gentle yoga class. Do not overdo it with high-intensity training or weight training until you are past the two-week mark. If you have access to an infrared sauna, that would be great to use during your program and allow you to sweat without putting stress on your adrenal glands. Aim for twenty minutes in the infrared sauna, and be sure to hydrate and include electrolytes after sauna use.

THE 30-DAY MEAL PLAN

Here are a few things to keep in mind with your meal plan to help you achieve the most success:

The meal plan is a sample of what 30 days on the Hormone Solution would look like. You can choose from any of the recipes in this book and create your own 30-day plan.

Your meal plan does not include leftovers, as I created your plan so you can see the variety of food and meals to include over a 30-day period. That said, leftovers are encouraged, as this will help you use up any food and prevent waste. And let's face it, who makes a new meal every day for breakfast, lunch and dinner? Keep it simple and reuse recipes.

I always encourage variety as much as possible, but there is nothing wrong with eating the same breakfast, lunch and dinner three days in a row. If this is what suits your schedule and needs, then go for it.

You won't find the elixirs on your meal plan, but feel free to include them throughout the day *with your meals*, maybe the Coconut Collagen Coffee (page 162) with your breakfast, or the Anti-Inflammatory Turmeric Latte (page 158) with your lunch. These are extras you can enjoy alongside your meals.

I encourage you to keep the treats to a minimum. I've included delicious grain-free desserts you can enjoy throughout your reset. For optimal results, keep desserts out of your diet for the first two weeks. Afterward, go ahead and introduce them, limiting them to one or two servings a week. If you're looking for some extra gut-healing support, include two or three Gut Gummies (page 204) with one of your meals.

If you don't feel satiated by a meal or you feel too full, feel free to add or take away from a recipe. For example, if a bowl of soup doesn't seem like enough for you, include a salad or a protein on the side.

I want you to know there is no right or wrong way to go about this. Feel like eating a bowl of soup alongside your dinner? Go for it. Feel like fasting in the morning and starting your day with a Coconut Collagen Coffee? Do it.

I want you to tune into your body and what it wants and needs. Let's get out of the diet mentality, and let's ditch counting calories or obsessing over macros. Count nutrients. Eat whole foods. Don't overeat. Pay attention to hunger. Drink enough water. You got this!

Last, don't overcomplicate it. It's all about the big picture here. It's not just about meal by meal, but what you do consistently over a 30-day period—and beyond—that is really going to shift your hormones and health.

YOUR 3-DAY LIQUID CLEANSE

It's time to begin your reset! Your first three days will begin with a liquid cleanse. No, you won't be consuming just water; you'll be enjoying delicious smoothies and soups throughout the three days that will help flood your body with potent nutrients.

Feel free to pick from any of the smoothie or soup recipes in this book. Repeat the recipes daily to keep it easy and use up leftovers, or feel free to make something new every day. It's your call!

If you feel hungry, go ahead and include an apple, pear or ½ cup (about 75 g) of berries with your soup, but be sure to have the fruit with your meal and not as a snack. Aim for a roughly five-hour break between your meals.

Be sure to get in 3 liters (12.5 cups) of water a day, and be sure to eat enough soup until you feel satiated.

Important note: Start each morning with a warm glass of water, a squeeze of lemon juice and ½ tablespoon (8 ml) of apple cider vinegar OR enjoy 1 cup (240 ml) of warm bone broth.

DAY	BREAKFAST	LUNCH	DINNER
1	Sweet Greens Smoothie, page 150	The Bieler Broth, page 170	Sweet Potato Soup, page 169
2	Chocolate Cherry Bomb Smoothie, page 146	The Bieler Broth	Sweet Potato Soup
3	Mint Chocolate Chip Smoothie, page 145	The Bieler Broth	Sweet Potato Soup

DAY	BREAKFAST	LUNCH	DINNER
4	Stuffed Avocado & Salmon Boats, page 103	Creamy Cauliflower "No Potato" Salad, page 198, with a slice of Grain-Free Almond Flour Bread, page 100	Meatloaf Muffins, page 127, with Broccoli Rice, page 197
5	Chocolate Cherry Bomb Smoothie, page 146	The Best Cobb Salad, page 174	Dijon-Dill Herbed Wild Salmon, page 139, + Berry Kale Salad, page 177
6	Raspberry Chia Pudding, page 112	Paleo Taco Bowl, page 124	Chicken and Tomato Instant Pot Stew, page 132, + Garlicky Cauliflower Rice, page 194
7	Breakfast Patties, page 107	Healing Chicken Soup, page 166	Korean Beef Short Ribs, page 115, + Roasted Asparagus, page 190
8	Pumpkin Pie Smoothie, page 149	Cast-Iron Roasted Chicken Thighs with Veggies, page 128	Sweet Potato, Beet & Arugula Detox Salad, page 181, + Roasted Turkey Thighs, page 136
9	On-the-Go Veggie Egg Cups, page 108	Creamy Cauliflower Soup, page 173	Lemon Dijon Chicken Thighs, page 120, + Shaved Brussels Sprouts with Bacon & Walnuts, page 193
10	Mint Chocolate Chip Smoothie, page 145	Whole Roasted Cauliflower with Za'atar Ghee, page 201, + Turmeric Turkey with Wilted Greens, page 116	Paleo Chili, page 131
11	Overnight No'Oats, page 111	Lamb Burgers with Plantain Fries, page 135	Baked Sea Bass with Pineapple Salsa, page 140, + Herbed Roasted Sweet Potatoes, page 189
12	Sweet Greens Smoothie, page 150	Paleo Taco Bowl, page 124	Cast-Iron Chicken Thighs with Veggies, page 128

DAY	BREAKFAST	LUNCH	DINNER
13	Stuffed Avocado & Salmon Boats, page 103	The Bieler Broth, page 170, + side serving of Berry Kale Salad, page 177	Garlic Shrimp with Walnut Pesto Zoodles, page 143
14	Chocolate Cherry Bomb Smoothie, page 146	Healing Chicken Soup, page 166	Lamb Burgers with Plantain Fries, page 135
15	Grain-Free Protein-Packed Crepes, page 99	Sweet Potato, Beet & Arugula Detox Salad, page 181, + Roasted Turkey Thighs, page 136	Baked Sea Bass with Pineapple Salsa, page 140, + Whole Roasted Cauliflower with Za'atar Ghee, page 201
16	Breakfast Patties, page 107	The Best Cobb Salad, page 174	Dijon-Dill Herbed Wild Salmon, page 139, + Avocado, Tomato & Cucumber Salad, page 178
17	On-the-Go Veggie Egg Cups, page 108	Shaved Brussels Sprouts with Bacon & Walnuts, page 193, + Chinese Ginger Chicken, page 119	Cauliflower Gnocchi with Homemade Roasted Cherry Tomato Sauce + your choice of protein, page 202
18	Avocado Toast with Eggs, page 104	Creamy Cauliflower Soup, page 173	Meatloaf Muffins, page 127, + Broccoli Rice, page 197
19	Overnight No'Oats, page 111	Dijon-Dill Herbed Wild Salmon, page 139, + Roasted Asparagus, page 190	Turmeric Turkey with Wilted Greens, page 116, + Shaved Brussels Sprouts with Bacon and Walnuts, page 193
20	Mint Chocolate Chip Smoothie, page 145	Roasted Asparagus, page 190, + Lemon Dijon Chicken Thighs, page 120	Korean Beef Short Ribs, page 115, + Berry Kale Salad, page 177
21	Grain-Free Protein-Packed Crepes, page 99	The Bieler Broth, page 170 + your choice of side salad	Garlic Shrimp with Walnut Pesto Zoodles, page 143

(continued)

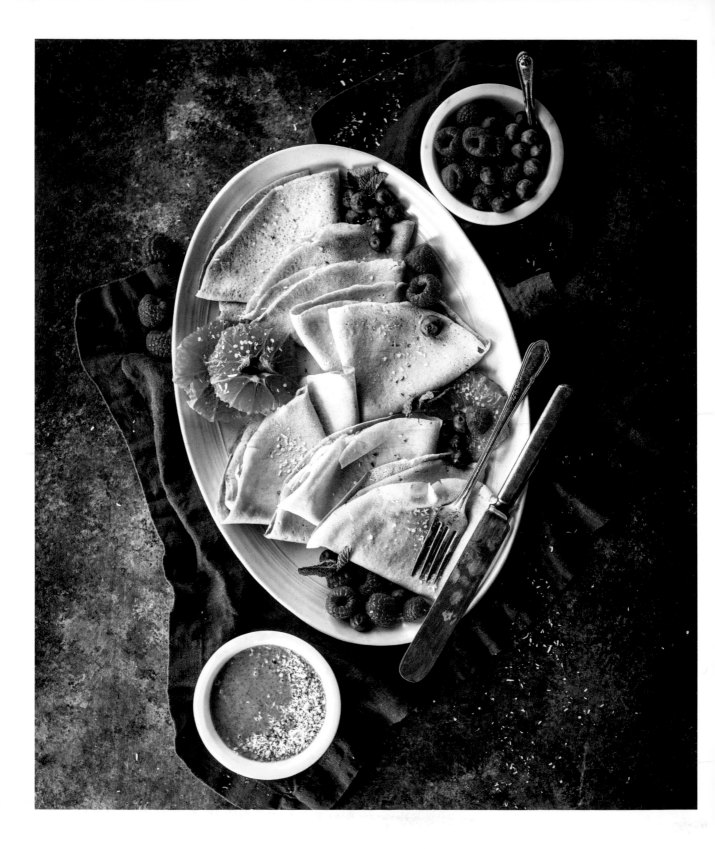

DAY	BREAKFAST	LUNCH	DINNER
22	Raspberry Chia Pudding, page 112	Paleo Chili, page 131	Dijon-Dill Herbed Wild Salmon, page 139, + Whole Roasted Cauliflower with Za'atar Ghee, page 201
23	Chocolate Cherry Bomb Smoothie, page 146	Sheet-Pan Chicken Stir-Fry, page 123	Avocado, Tomato & Cucumber Salad, page 178, + Meatloaf Muffins, page 127
24	Breakfast Patties, page 107	Baked Sea Bass with Pineapple Salsa, page 140, + Broccoli Rice, page 197	Shaved Brussels Sprouts with Bacon & Walnuts, page 193, + Chinese Ginger Chicken, page 119
25	On-the-Go Veggie Egg Cups, page 108	Cauliflower Gnocchi with Homemade Roasted Cherry Tomato Sauce + your choice of protein, page 202	Paleo Taco Bowl, page 124
26	Overnight No'Oats, page 111	Avocado, Tomato & Cucumber Salad, page 178, + Turmeric Turkey with Wilted Greens, page 116	Meatloaf Muffins, page 127, + Roasted Asparagus, page 190
27	Sweet Greens Smoothie, page 150	Lamb Burgers with Plantain Fries, page 135	Sheet-Pan Chicken Stir-Fry, page 123
28	Avocado Toast with Eggs, page 104	Sweet Potato Soup, page 169	Korean Beef Short Ribs, page 115, + Garlicky Cauliflower Rice, page 194
29	Stuffed Avocado & Salmon Boats, page 103	Paleo Taco Bowl, page 124	Chicken and Tomato Instant Pot Stew, page 132
30	Pumpkin Pie Smoothie, page 149	Breakfast Patties, page 107	Sweet Potato, Beet & Arugula Detox Salad, page 181, + Roasted Turkey Thighs, page 136

PART 3:
RECIPES

GRAIN-FREE PROTEIN-PACKED CREPES

Whether you like sweet or savory, these crepes can work either way! I often fill mine with sautéed mushrooms, spinach and a bit of sauerkraut. Or try almond butter and a mix of fresh berries. Either version is a delicious, hearty and protein-packed way to start your day.

MAKES 4 TO 6 CREPES

4 eggs

1 cup (240 ml) unsweetened coconut milk

½ cup (60 g) tapioca flour

½ cup (51 g) almond flour

½ tsp baking powder

½ tsp ground cinnamon

Pinch of sea salt

Coconut oil, for greasing pan

Combine the eggs, coconut milk, tapioca flour, almond flour, baking powder, cinnamon and sea salt in a large bowl. Whisk them together until smooth. A few lumps may remain, which is okay. Heat a small amount of coconut oil in a skillet or crepe pan over medium heat.

Add the batter to the pan using a soup ladle or ¼-cup (60-ml) measuring cup, tilting the pan gently to evenly spread out the batter. You want a thin layer covering your pan. It's like making a pancake, but a thin and large pancake! Cook until the edges start to set, then gently flip it and cook on the other side for about 1 to 2 minutes.

Transfer the fresh crepe onto a plate or wire rack to cool, or eat it right away while still warm. Make the remaining crepes with the batter, and spread on your favorite toppings!

*See photo on page 96.

GRAIN-FREE ALMOND FLOUR BREAD

Back in my teenage years, English muffins and toast were staples for breakfast. Slather on some peanut butter and jam, and you're golden! I used to think I was doing a good thing for my body, but an hour later I was left starving! Hello, irregular blood sugar. This grain-free almond bread is delicious, and it can be made sweet or savory or left just as is. Feel free to add some cinnamon or ground vanilla bean for a sweeter option. Or try a more savory bread by adding in dried herbs, such as thyme or rosemary.

SERVES 8

Coconut oil, for greasing pan
3½ cups (333 g) almond flour
¾ tsp baking soda
¼ tsp sea salt
4 large eggs
1 tbsp (15 ml) raw honey
¾ tsp apple cider vinegar

Preheat the oven to 300°F (150°C, or gas mark 2), and grease a loaf pan.

Combine the almond flour, baking soda and sea salt in a large bowl. In a separate bowl, whisk together the eggs, then add the honey and apple cider vinegar. Whisk to combine them.

Pour the wet ingredients into the dry and stir them together. Pour the batter into the loaf pan. Bake the bread for 45 minutes, until it is golden-brown and a toothpick inserted in the center comes out clean.

NOTE: Slice the bread when cooled. If you are not using it right away, place it in the freezer. Then just grab a slice as you need it. I've paired this bread with the Creamy Cauliflower "No Potato" Salad recipe (page 198) for a hearty lunch or dinner. It's also great alongside the Chicken and Tomato Instant Pot Stew (page 132) or Paleo Chili (page 131).

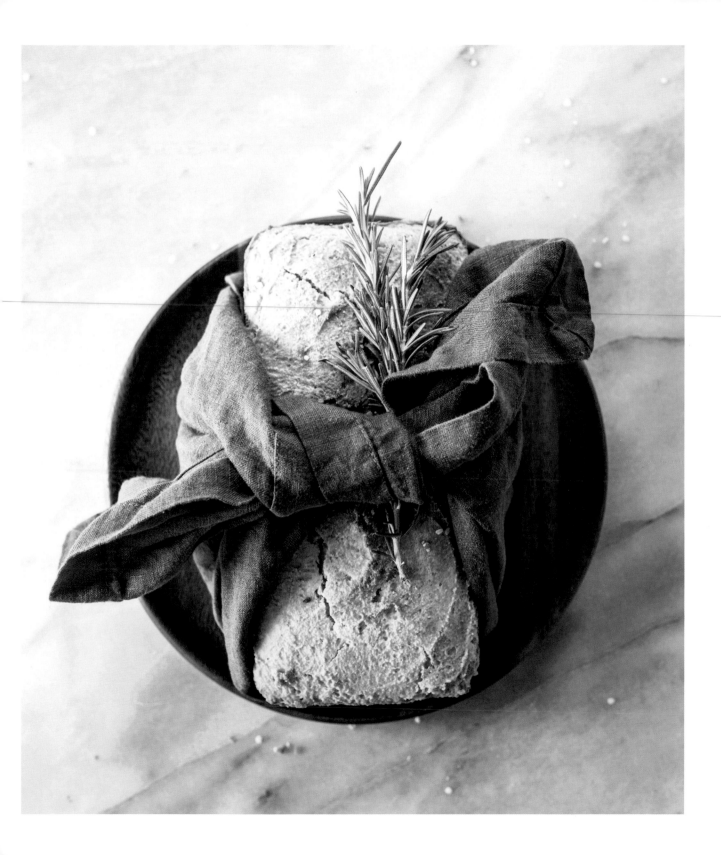

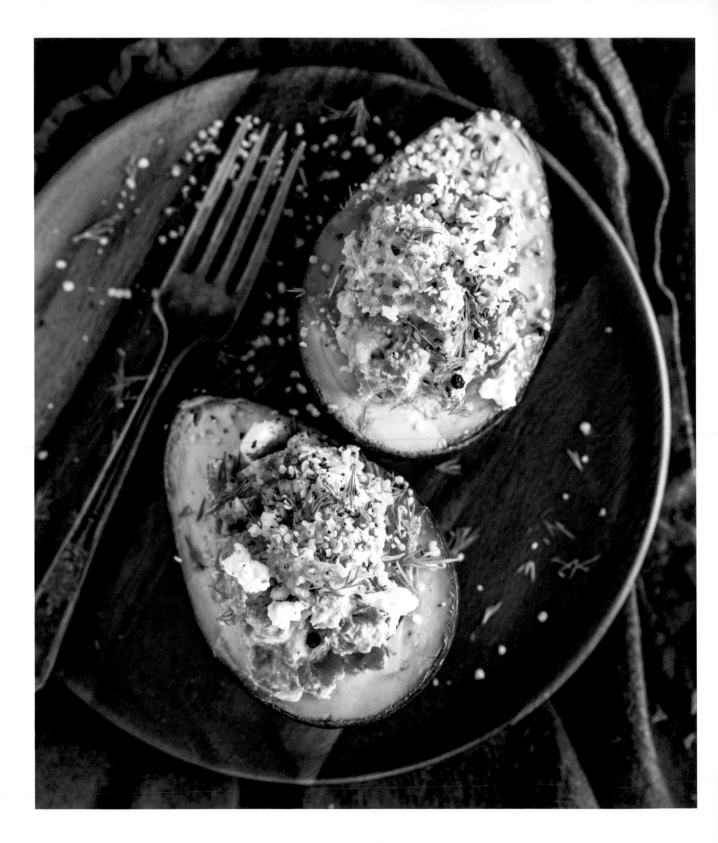

STUFFED AVOCADO & SALMON BOATS

Your body craves protein and fat at breakfast. These two macronutrients will keep you full and stoke your metabolism. I absolutely love the combo of avocado and salmon together. This hearty and savory breakfast will provide you with a ton of energy, balance your blood sugar and, as a bonus, provide you with anti-aging omega-3s and vitamin E.

SERVES 1

1 medium ripe avocado

2–3 slices wild-caught smoked salmon

1 oz (28 g) fresh, soft goat or sheep cheese (optional)

2 tbsp (30 ml) olive oil

Juice of 1 lemon

1 tsp Herbamare seasoning

Pinch of sea salt

Hemp seeds, for garnish

Slice the avocado in half and remove the seed. Using a spoon, gently remove the avocado from the skin. Set it aside.

In a small food processor, pulse together the smoked salmon, cheese (if using), olive oil, lemon juice, seasoning and sea salt.

Place the salmon mixture inside the avocado, and sprinkle on the hemp seeds.

AVOCADO TOAST WITH EGGS

Sometimes, the easiest of ingredients come together to make a perfect and healthy meal, like this recipe! It's so simple and delicious. I love to enjoy this breakfast on a Sunday morning with a cup of herbal tea. It's satiating and fuels me for a day of doing nothing—Sundays are typically my do-nothing day! If one slice and one egg are satiating enough, go with that.

SERVES 1

2 slices Grain-Free Almond Flour Bread (page 100)

½ avocado

¼ tsp dried oregano

¼ tsp Herbamare seasoning

2 eggs, poached, fried or scrambled

½ tbsp (7 g) grass-fed butter or coconut oil

Pinch of sea salt

Toast the almond bread. While the bread is toasting, mash the avocado with the dried oregano and seasoning. Set it aside. Prepare the eggs to your liking.

Spread the butter on the warm toast. Top it with the mashed avocado and an egg, and sprinkle on some sea salt.

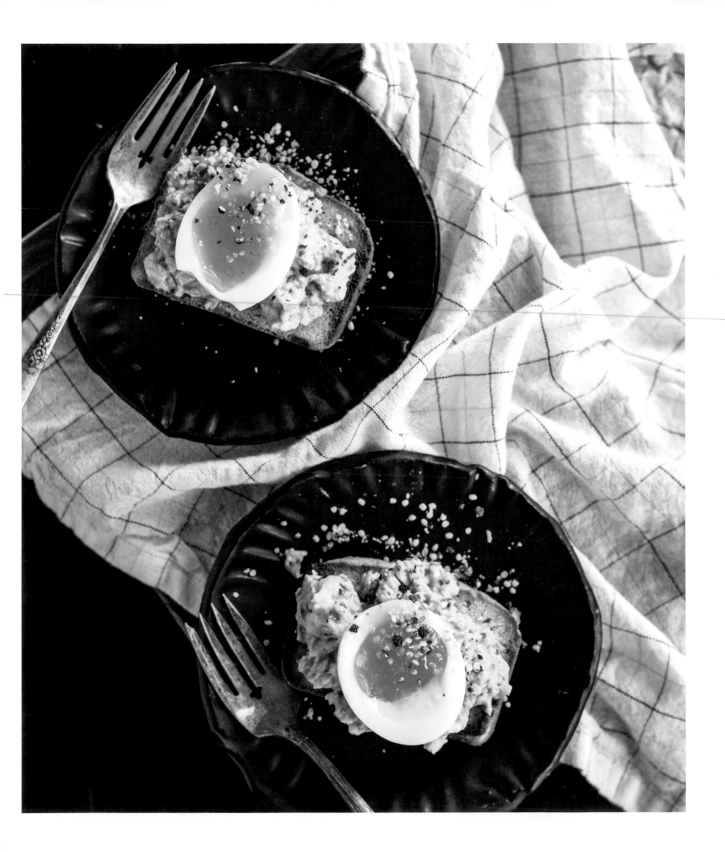

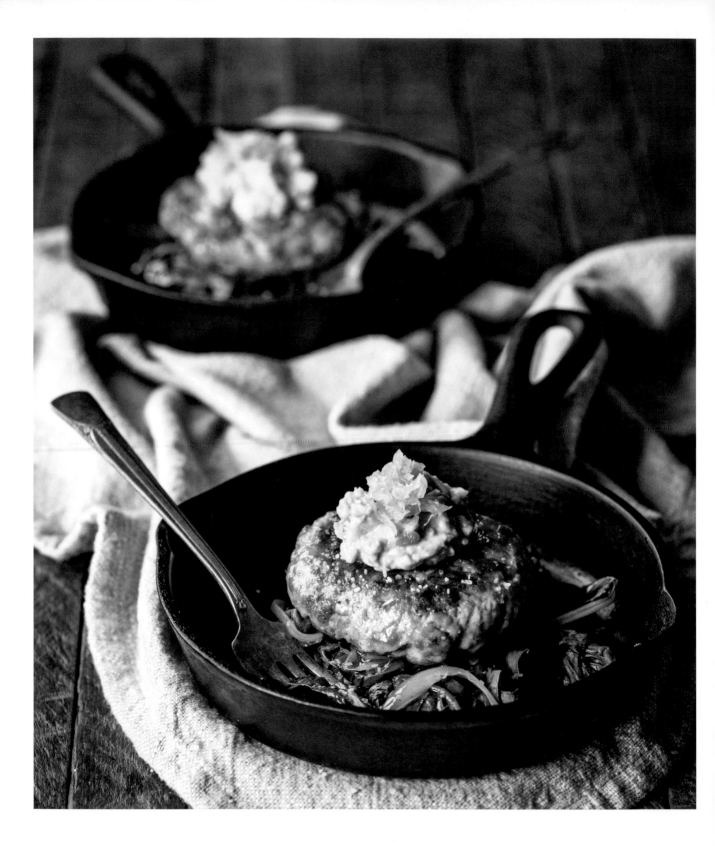

BREAKFAST PATTIES

Homemade breakfast sausages are easier to make than you think. Having these on hand for a quick grab-and-go breakfast will ensure you are getting in enough metabolism-boosting protein first thing in the morning. I often use the Primal Palate Breakfast Blend seasoning mix, but I've listed out the herbs individually in this recipe. Pair these patties with some sautéed greens plus a serving of mashed avocado, for a delicious and savory breakfast.

SERVES 4

1 lb (454 g) ground pork or turkey

1 tsp fennel

1 tsp garlic powder

1 tsp paprika

½ tsp sage

½ tsp sea salt

¼ tsp cayenne pepper

¼ tsp white pepper

3 tbsp (40 g) coconut oil or other cooking oil, divided

2 shallots, sliced

3 cups (90 g) fresh spinach

1 small avocado, mashed

3–4 tbsp (27–36 g) sauerkraut

Combine the pork with the fennel, garlic powder, paprika, sage, sea salt, cayenne pepper and white pepper in a mixing bowl. Using your hands, mix everything together until well incorporated, then shape the mixture into four patties.

Heat a large skillet over medium heat, and add 2 tablespoons (27 g) of coconut oil. Cook the patties for about 5 to 7 minutes per side. Each side should be golden, and the center of the patties should no longer be pink. When cooked through, remove the patties from the pan and set them aside.

Add the remaining 1 tablespoon (13 g) of oil with the shallots. Cook for 1 minute, then add the spinach. Cook until the spinach is soft and wilted, about 3 to 4 minutes.

Serve the patties over the wilted spinach with a dollop of mashed avocado and sauerkraut.

ON-THE-GO VEGGIE EGG CUPS

This is a no-excuse morning recipe that you can whip up the night before and have ready to grab and go the next morning. Eggs provide incredible protein and are loaded with minerals such as selenium, zinc, iron and copper—all essential nutrients needed for optimal hormonal health. If you can tolerate dairy, feel free to add some crumbled goat or sheep feta into the egg mixture after you've poured it into the muffin pan.

MAKES 6

Coconut oil or ghee, for greasing pan

1 red bell pepper, diced

4 cherry tomatoes, diced

3 spring onions, chopped

1 handful of spinach, kale or arugula, roughly chopped

6 large eggs

1 tsp dried oregano

1 tsp dried basil

½ tsp red pepper flakes or a few splashes of your favorite hot sauce (optional)

½ tsp sea salt

3 tbsp (27 g) your favorite sauerkraut or kimchi, for serving

Preheat the oven to 375°F (190°C, or gas mark 5), and grease a 6-cup muffin tin with coconut oil. Set it aside.

In a large bowl, add the bell pepper, tomatoes, onions and spinach. Add the eggs, oregano, basil, red pepper flakes (if using) and sea salt. Whisk together until they're well combined. Gently pour the egg mixture evenly into the 6 muffin cups.

Place the tray in the oven and bake for 18 to 20 minutes, or until the egg cups are cooked through. If you prefer a crisper egg cup, bake for roughly 25 minutes. Serve with the sauerkraut alongside.

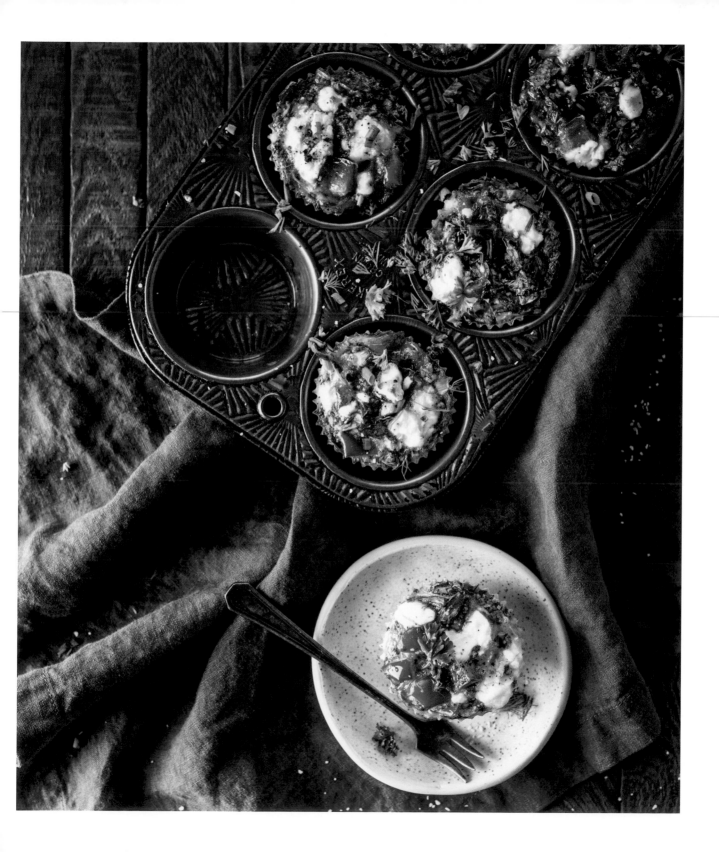

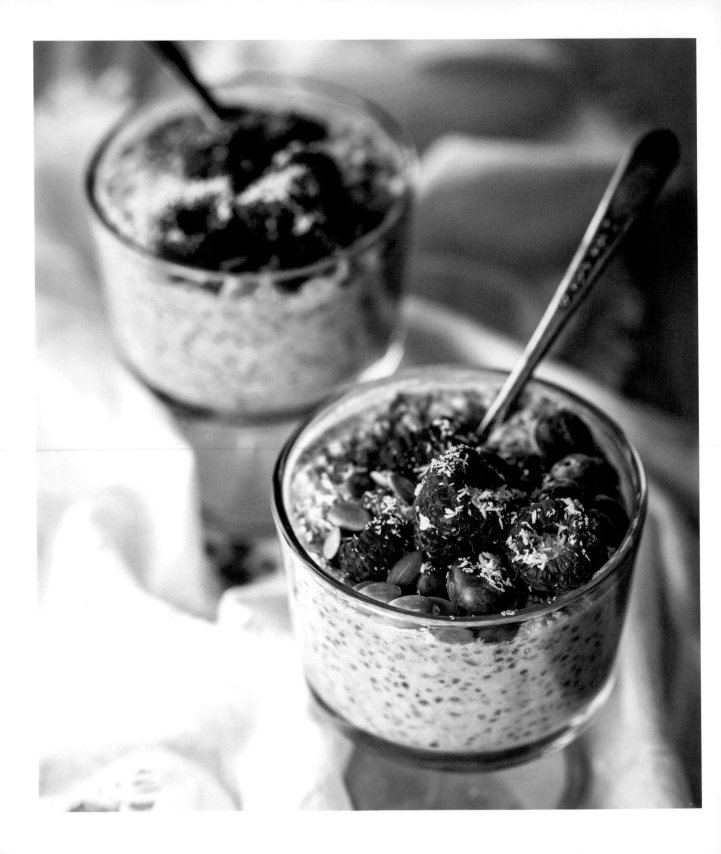

OVERNIGHT NO'OATS

I used to love oatmeal, and I still do. But since grains are no longer a staple in my diet, I was on a mission to find an alternative. I absolutely love this recipe. Make it the night before and you're all set for a busy morning when you're in a rush. You can also double the recipe, divide it up into jars, top it with fruit and no morning prep is needed—so no excuses now! This recipe is quite filling due to the high fat content from the nuts. I also love mixing in some collagen powder for the added protein boost.

SERVES 2

1¼ cups (weight will vary) nuts (I like a combination of walnuts, pecans, pili nuts, sunflower seeds or pumpkin seeds)

2 tbsp (20 g) chia seeds

1½ tsp (6 g) ground flaxseeds

1 tbsp (15 ml) maple syrup

½ tsp vanilla extract

½ tsp ground cinnamon

Pinch of sea salt

1½ cups (360 ml) coconut milk

TOPPING IDEAS

Fresh or frozen berries

Shredded coconut

Nut butter

Raw cacao nibs

Scoop of collagen powder

In a food processor, pulse the nuts until they are grainy and crumbled. Then transfer them to a large mason jar. Add the chia seeds, flaxseeds, maple syrup, vanilla, cinnamon, sea salt and coconut milk to the jar. Stir to combine everything, or seal it with the lid and give it a really good shake. Cover and place it in the fridge overnight.

In the morning, remove the jar from the fridge. Pour the no'oats into a serving bowl, or heat it up on the stovetop. Add your favorite toppings and serve.

RASPBERRY CHIA PUDDING

Nothing beats waking up in the morning to an already-made breakfast! I suggest making this the night before so it's ready to go in the morning, but it will be just fine made on the spot. This delicious chia pudding is full of antioxidants and fiber to keep you fueled and energized for your morning. Feel free to top it with nuts, seeds, shredded coconut or your favorite superfoods.

SERVES 1

1 cup (240 ml) almond or coconut milk

1 cup (123 g) fresh or frozen raspberries, divided

1 tsp pure vanilla extract or vanilla stevia

1 tsp ground cinnamon

Juice of ½ lemon

3 tbsp (30 g) chia seeds

Shaved chocolate, for serving (optional)

In a food processor or blender, combine the almond milk, ½ cup (62 g) of the raspberries, vanilla, cinnamon and lemon juice. Process together until it's smooth.

Pour the mixture into a mason jar, and add the chia seeds. Put the lid on and give it a good shake to incorporate the chia. Let it rest for 1 hour or in the refrigerator overnight. Shake the jar a few times to help combine them. Pour the pudding into a bowl, and top it with the remaining raspberries.

Alternatively, you can serve this chia pudding right away. For a more decadent treat, enjoy this at night with shaved chocolate on top.

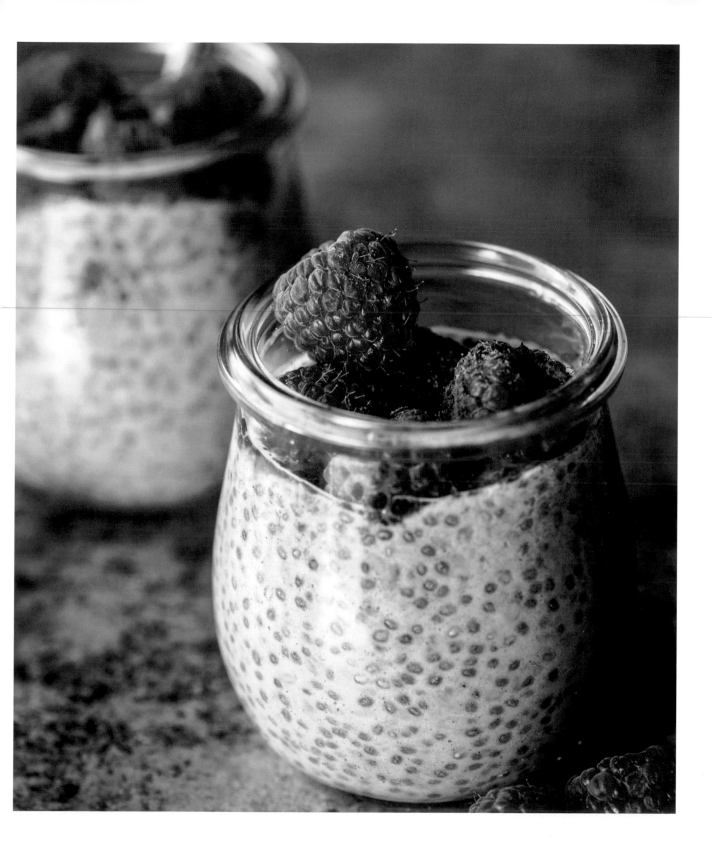

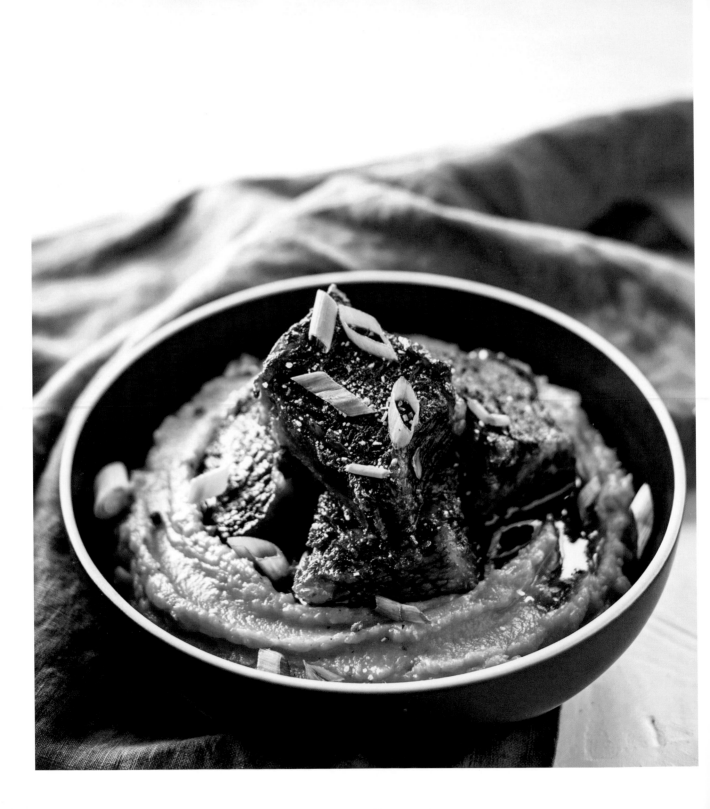

MAINS

KOREAN BEEF SHORT RIBS

Weeknight meals are a breeze now that the Instant Pot® has come into my life. These Korean beef short ribs are fall-off-the-bone delicious, and the marinade takes all of five minutes to whip up. Throw it all in your Instant Pot, set it and forget it. And in no time, you have what looks like a gourmet meal. Be sure to purchase organic and pasture-raised meat. This is key for hormonal health, plus you'll be eating higher amounts of anti-inflammatory omega-3s, which is great for your heart, skin and gut.

SERVES 4

5 lb (2.3 kg) bone-in short ribs, English-style cut (If using a 6-quart [6-L] Instant Pot, don't go above 5 lb [2.3 kg] or it won't all fit.)

2 tsp (6 g) sea salt

¼ tsp black pepper

2 tbsp (30 ml) avocado oil

Garlicky Cauliflower Rice (page 194), Whole Roasted Cauliflower with Za'atar Ghee (page 201) or mashed sweet potatoes, for serving

MARINADE

½ cup (120 ml) coconut aminos

½ cup (120 ml) bone broth

1 tbsp (15 ml) apple cider vinegar

2 tsp (10 ml) fish sauce

1 large Asian pear or Fuji apple, roughly chopped

6 cloves garlic, roughly chopped

3 green onions (green and white part), roughly chopped

2-inch (5-cm) piece of fresh ginger, roughly chopped

½ tbsp (8 ml) hot sauce (optional)

Small handful of roughly chopped fresh cilantro (optional)

Place the short ribs in a large bowl, and season them with the sea salt and pepper. Heat a cast-iron pan over medium heat. Add the avocado oil, and brown the short ribs on each side for 3 to 4 minutes. You may need to do this in batches, using more oil with each batch.

Turn on the Instant Pot. As you finish browning the ribs, add them to the pot. You may have to play Tetris to get all the ribs to fit.

When all the ribs are browned and added to the pot, start on the marinade. In a food processor, add the coconut aminos, broth, vinegar, fish sauce, pear, garlic, onions, fresh ginger, hot sauce (if using) and cilantro (if using). Blend until they're well combined. Pour the marinade over the ribs. Using your hands, gently mix the marinade into the ribs, making sure enough liquid reaches the bottom of the pot.

Hit Manual on your Instant Pot, and set the timer for 45 minutes. It will take time for the ribs to come to pressure. When 45 minutes is up, be sure to let the pressure naturally release for at least 15 to 20 minutes before releasing it yourself and opening the lid. Serve over cauliflower rice, za'atar roasted cauliflower or mashed sweet potatoes.

TURMERIC TURKEY WITH WILTED GREENS

I love whipping up some turmeric turkey when I'm strapped for time. Turkey is a great source of protein, and I've combined it with some powerful anti-inflammatory spices. Serve this recipe alongside some Broccoli Rice (page 197) or Garlicky Cauliflower Rice (page 194), Herbed Roasted Sweet Potatoes (page 189) or a slice of Grain-Free Almond Flour Bread (page 100) as a sloppy Joe. As a note, you can replace the turkey with ground beef, lamb or chicken.

SERVES 2 TO 3

2 tbsp (30 ml) olive oil, ghee or other cooking oil

1 lb (454 g) ground white or dark turkey meat

½ cup (120 ml) chicken broth, divided

1 tsp onion powder

1 tsp garlic powder

½ tsp dried coriander

2 tsp (4 g) turmeric

¼ tsp cumin

¼ tsp cayenne pepper

½ tsp salt

4 cups (120 g) fresh spinach or kale, roughly chopped

Heat a skillet over medium heat. Add the oil and the turkey meat. Break the turkey up into chunks using a spatula. Add ¼ cup (60 ml) of broth along with the onion powder, garlic powder, coriander, turmeric, cumin, cayenne pepper and salt.

Continue to break up the turkey into small pieces as you stir all the ingredients together. Cook for 6 to 8 minutes, then add the remaining ¼ cup (60 ml) of chicken broth, along with the spinach. Cook for another 4 minutes, until the turkey meat is cooked through and the greens have wilted.

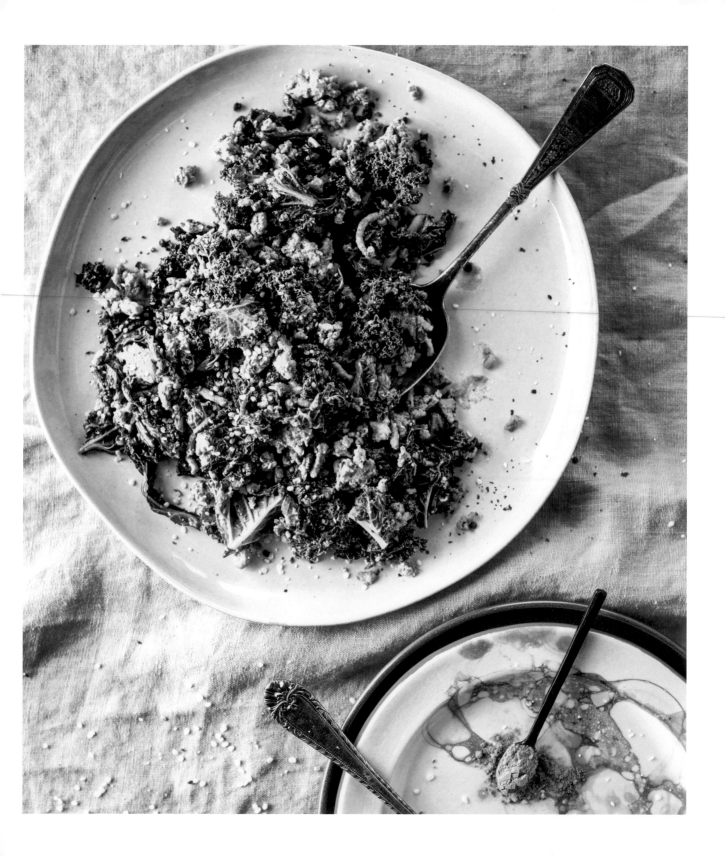

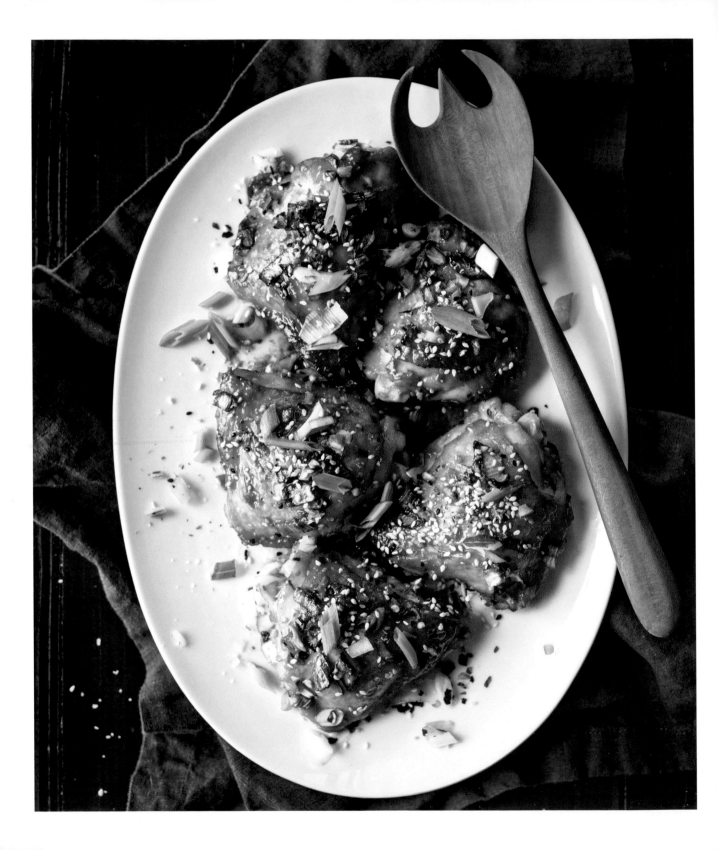

CHINESE GINGER CHICKEN

This recipe has become a favorite in our home. It's simple to make and requires only a handful of ingredients—and it tastes amazing! It's definitely better than any Chinese take-out you'll ever have, plus it's healthier. You can use ground ginger in this recipe, but fresh ginger lends much more flavor. Ginger is one of my favorite anti-inflammatory herbs. It's great for nausea and joint pain, and it's ideal to consume during cold and flu season.

SERVES 3 TO 4

6–8 bone-in skin-on chicken thighs

1 medium red onion, chopped

2 cloves garlic, minced

2 tsp (4 g) minced fresh ginger

1 tsp onion powder

2 tsp (5 g) sesame seeds

1 tsp red pepper flakes

⅓ cup (80 ml) coconut aminos

Sea salt and pepper

Preheat the oven to 350°F (175°C, or gas mark 4).

In a large bowl, add the chicken, onion, garlic, fresh ginger, onion powder, sesame seeds, red pepper flakes, coconut aminos, sea salt and pepper. Mix them together well.

Place the chicken thighs on a baking sheet lined with parchment paper. Cook for 35 minutes (if you're using boneless, skinless thighs, cook for 25 to 30 minutes). Turn the broiler to low and cook for 5 to 10 minutes, until the skin is nice and brown. Remove and serve them hot.

DIRECTIONS FOR THE INSTANT POT:

Add the chicken, onion, garlic, ginger, onion powder, sesame seeds, red pepper flakes, coconut aminos, sea salt and pepper to the Instant Pot. Give it a quick stir to help distribute the marinade and coat the chicken. Make sure the liquid has reached the bottom of the pot. Hit Manual on your Instant Pot, and set the timer for 15 minutes. If you're using boneless, skinless chicken thighs, set the timer for 10 minutes. When the timer is done, manually release the pressure.

LEMON DIJON CHICKEN THIGHS

This recipe is on a weekly rotation in our house because it's THAT good and it's so easy to make. As a bonus, the marinade works great on salmon as well. If you're ever stuck in a "what do I make for dinner rut," make this recipe. I promise it will win over the hearts of grown-ups and little ones. If you are purchasing organic chicken, you can leave the skin on. There are lots of healthy fats in the skin, but it's only okay to eat if it's organic and pasture raised. Serve this with a side of Roasted Asparagus (page 190) or a large salad for a simple and healthy weeknight meal.

SERVES 4

8 organic chicken thighs, skin-on if organic

2 tbsp (30 ml) Dijon mustard

1 tbsp (15 g) grainy mustard

2 sprigs fresh rosemary, removed from sprigs and chopped

2 sprigs fresh thyme, removed from sprigs

2 tbsp (30 ml) olive oil

Juice of ½ lemon

Pinch of sea salt and fresh pepper

Preheat the oven to 350°F (175°C, or gas mark 4), and line a baking tray with parchment paper.

Place the chicken in a large bowl and add the Dijon mustard, grainy mustard, rosemary, thyme, olive oil, lemon juice, sea salt and pepper. Using your hands, mix together the chicken and marinade really well.

Place the bowl in the fridge and let it sit for 20 to 30 minutes to marinate. If you don't have time to marinate the chicken, that's okay. You can cook it right away with great results and flavor!

Place the chicken on the baking tray and cook for 35 minutes. Turn the oven to a low broil and cook for another 10 minutes, until the skin is nice and crispy and fully cooked through. Be sure to watch the chicken as it broils as you don't want it to burn. Some ovens broil faster than others.

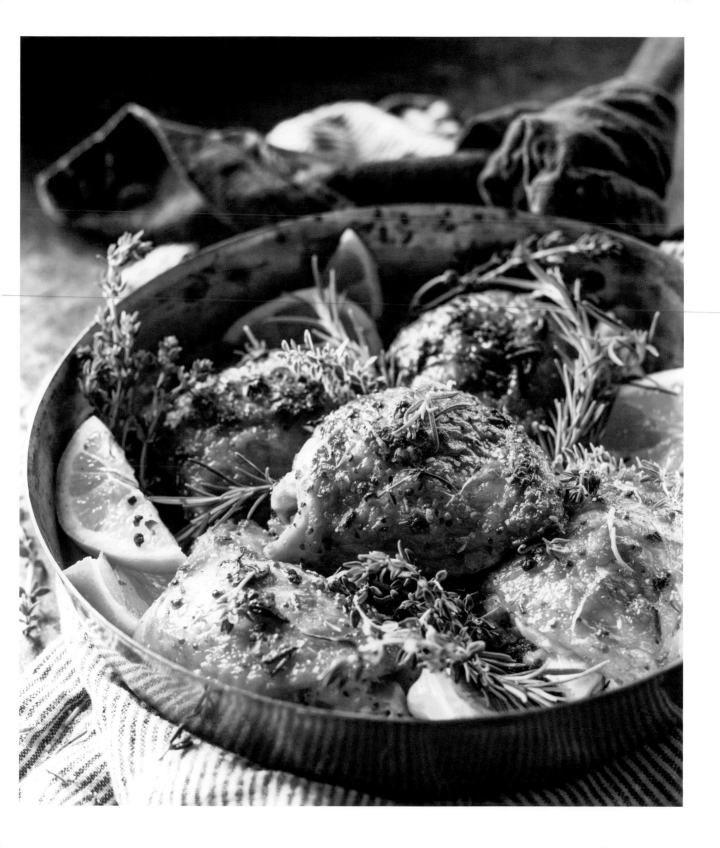

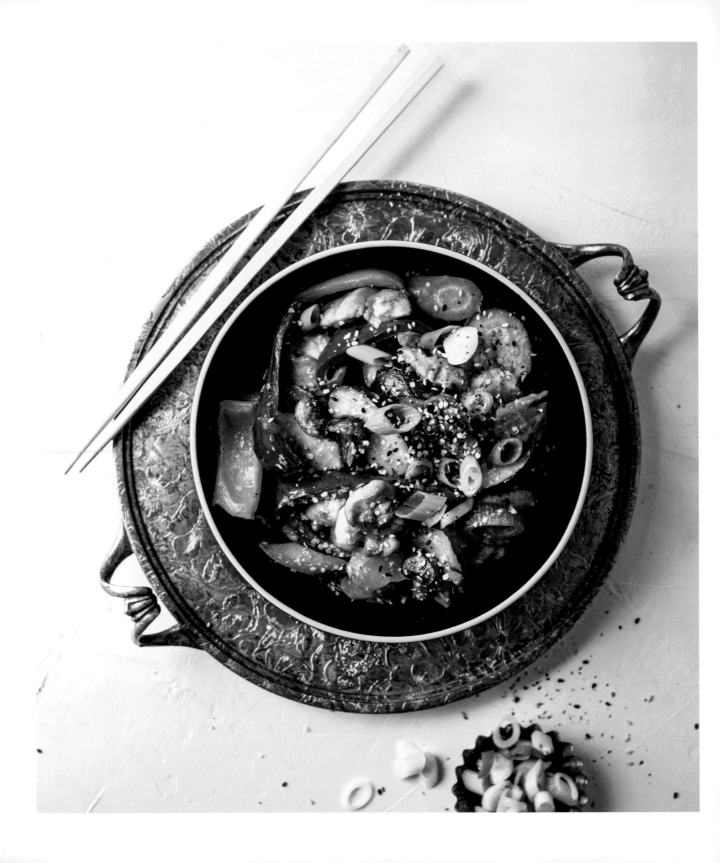

SHEET-PAN CHICKEN STIR-FRY

All hail sheet-pan dinners. Another meal that saves you time and cleanup. I often have this meal for breakfast and top it with a fried egg—oh so good!—because quality protein in the morning is the best way to support your metabolism and blood sugar. If you're feeling like chicken stir-fry leftovers for breakfast—go for it.

SERVES 4

FOR THE SAUCE

2 tbsp (30 ml) coconut aminos

1 tbsp (15 ml) rice vinegar (optional)

1 tbsp (15 ml) sesame oil

1 tbsp (8 g) minced garlic

½ tbsp (3 g) grated fresh ginger

1 tbsp (10 g) tapioca or arrowroot starch

FOR THE CHICKEN AND VEGGIES

1½ lb (680 g) boneless skinless chicken thighs, cut into 2-inch (5-cm) pieces

2 large carrots, peeled and cut diagonally into 2-inch (5-cm) pieces

1 small zucchini, cut diagonally into 2-inch (5-cm) pieces

2 red, green or yellow bell peppers, sliced

1 cup (70 g) mushrooms, sliced

½ red onion, sliced

Sprinkle of sesame seeds

2 green onions, roughly chopped

Preheat the oven to 400°F (200°C, or gas mark 6).

To make the sauce, whisk together the coconut aminos, rice vinegar (if using), sesame oil, garlic and fresh ginger. Slowly whisk in the tapioca starch 1 or 2 teaspoons (3 or 6 g) at a time to avoid any clumps. Set it aside.

To make the chicken and veggies, cover a baking sheet with parchment paper. Spread the chicken, carrots, zucchini, bell peppers, mushrooms and onion out on the baking sheet. Drizzle the sauce over the top. Using your hands or a spatula, combine everything together until all the chicken and vegetables are well coated with the sauce. Place the baking sheet in the oven and cook for 30 minutes, or until the chicken is fully cooked through. Sprinkle with sesame seeds and green onion just before serving.

PALEO TACO BOWL

This bowl is perfect for lunch or dinner, and I've often eaten the leftovers for breakfast. Between the cauliflower rice, beef and guac, you've got yourself a healthy balanced P+F+F (protein, fat and fiber) meal with a ton of flavor.

SERVES 2 TO 3

FOR THE CAULIFLOWER RICE

1 tbsp (14 g) coconut oil

12 oz (340 g) cauliflower rice

½ tsp sea salt

1 tbsp (15 ml) fresh lime juice

3 cloves garlic, chopped

1 tsp onion powder

Dash of chipotle powder

FOR THE BEEF

1 tbsp (14 g) coconut oil or other cooking fat

1 lb (454 g) grass-fed ground beef

1 small red onion, diced

½ tsp sea salt

¾ tsp onion powder

¾ tsp garlic powder

1 tsp cumin

¾ tsp chili powder

Chipotle powder, to taste

2 tbsp (32 g) tomato paste

¼ cup (60 ml) water or broth

FOR THE GUACAMOLE

1 large or 2 small ripe avocados, peeled, pitted and diced

2–3 tbsp (20–30 g) minced onion

1 clove garlic, minced

1½ tbsp (23 ml) fresh lime juice

½ tsp sea salt, or to taste

FOR THE TOPPINGS

2 cups (110 g) chopped romaine lettuce

1 tomato, diced

¼ cup (4 g) cilantro, roughly chopped (optional)

Additional lime juice and hot sauce, for serving (optional)

To make the cauliflower rice, heat a large skillet over medium heat. Add the coconut oil and riced cauliflower and stir to coat it. Add the sea salt, lime juice, garlic, onion powder and chipotle powder. Cover and cook for 5 to 6 minutes, then remove the skillet from the heat.

To make the beef, in a separate skillet, heat the coconut oil over medium-high heat. Add the beef to the skillet and break up large lumps with a wooden spoon or spatula. Add the onion, sea salt, onion powder, garlic powder, cumin, chili powder and chipotle powder. Cook, stirring occasionally, until the beef is browned and no longer pink. Do not drain the fat. Lower the heat to medium-low, add the tomato paste and water, and stir to combine them. Continue to cook and stir until it's thickened, then remove it to a separate bowl.

To make the guacamole, in a bowl, mash together the avocado with the onion, garlic, lime juice and sea salt. Adjust the seasoning to taste.

To assemble the bowls, place the cauliflower rice at the bottom of the bowl, then layer on the beef. Add the romaine lettuce, tomato and guacamole. Garnish with cilantro, a squeeze of lime juice and some hot sauce, if using.

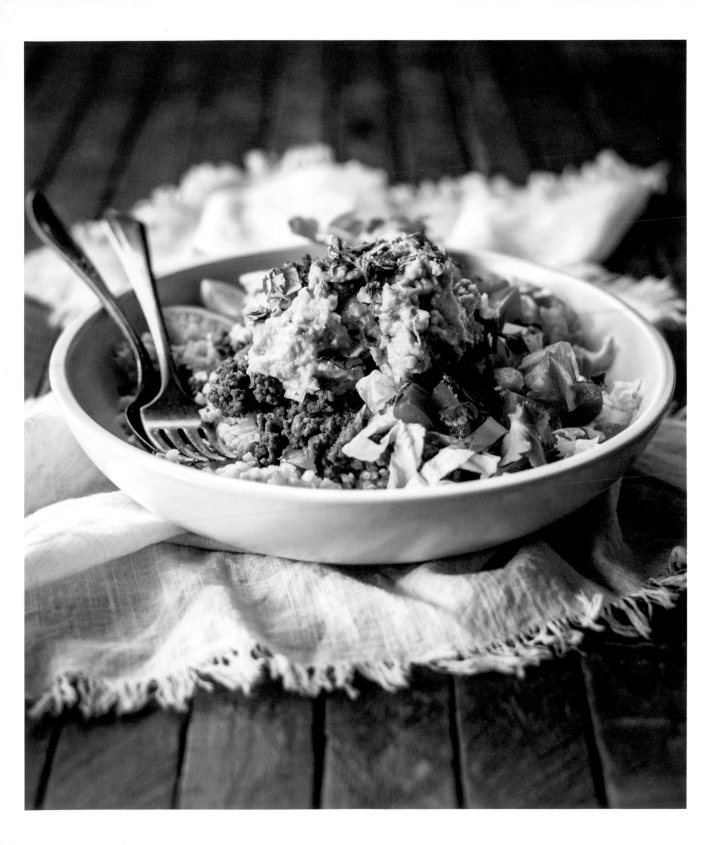

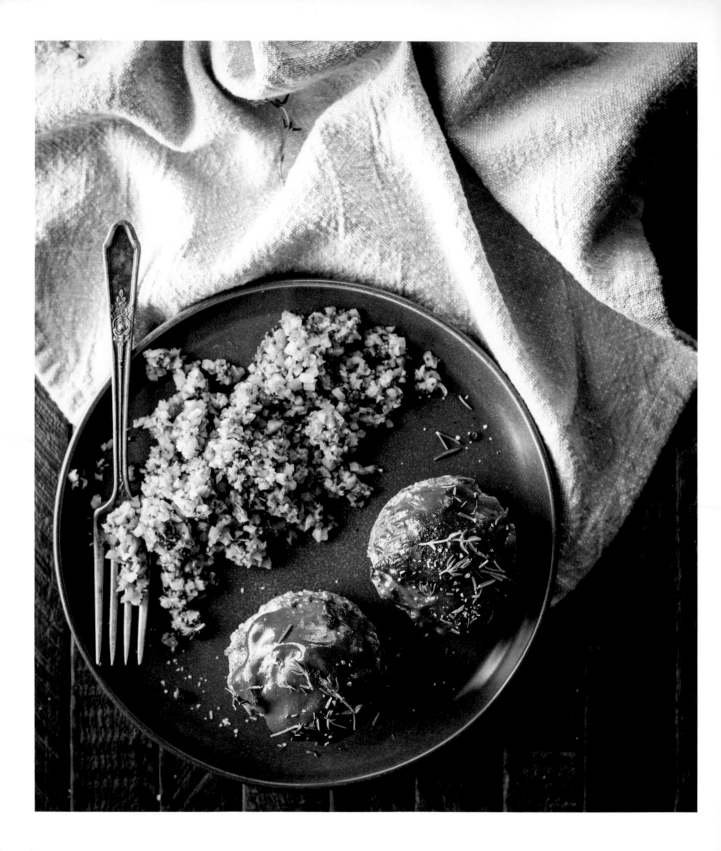

MEATLOAF MUFFINS

When we think of meatloaf, I feel that most of us don't get that excited. And then to combine it into a muffin? Trust me on this! This recipe is so damn good, and I know it's going to become a family staple. These are quick to make, perfect for leftovers the next day and they freeze well.

MAKES 12 MUFFINS

FOR THE MEAT MUFFINS

Olive oil or ghee, for greasing pan

2 eggs

1 (6-oz [170-g]) can of tomato paste

½ tbsp (3 g) dried oregano

1 tsp dried rosemary

1 tsp dried thyme

1 tsp sea salt

½ tbsp (8 ml) your favorite hot sauce

2 tbsp (30 ml) coconut aminos

2 lb (907 g) organic ground beef

¾ cup (120 g) chopped onion

FOR THE TOPPING

2 tbsp (18 g) coconut sugar

¼ cup (60 ml) ketchup

1 tbsp (15 ml) Dijon mustard

1 tbsp (15 g) prepared horseradish (optional)

Preheat the oven to 375°F (190°C, or gas mark 5). Lightly grease a 12-cup muffin pan with olive oil or ghee.

To make the muffins, in a large bowl, lightly whisk the eggs. Whisk in the tomato paste, oregano, rosemary, thyme, sea salt, hot sauce and coconut aminos. Add the ground beef and onion, and mix it all together thoroughly using your hands. Evenly mound the seasoned ground beef into the 12 muffin cups.

To make the topping, whisk together the sugar, ketchup, Dijon mustard and horseradish (if using) in a small bowl. Brush the topping evenly over the meaty muffin tops. Bake for 25 to 30 minutes, or until the muffins are cooked through.

NOTE: Serve this alongside Broccoli Rice (page 197) for a delicious weeknight meal.

CAST-IRON ROASTED CHICKEN THIGHS WITH VEGGIES

If you don't own a cast-iron pan, I highly recommend you purchase one. Being able to take the pan from stovetop to the oven is great. It's a one-pan meal, which also means less cleanup! And your stress hormones love less cleanup—amiright?!

SERVES 3

2 tbsp (30 ml) avocado oil, melted coconut oil or melted ghee

6 bone-in, skin-on chicken thighs

1 tsp dried thyme

1 tsp dried oregano

½ tsp sea salt

½ tsp black pepper

½ cup (120 ml) chicken broth or water

3 tbsp (45 ml) balsamic vinegar

2 cloves garlic, roughly chopped

½ onion, diced

2 small zucchini, diced

1 pint (298 g) cherry tomatoes

Cauliflower rice or a large green salad, for serving (optional)

Preheat the oven to 375°F (190°C, or gas mark 5).

Heat the oil in a large cast-iron pan over medium-high heat. When the oil is hot, add the chicken to the pan and brown the chicken on both sides, roughly 3 minutes per side. Season each side of the chicken with the thyme, oregano, sea salt and pepper as it is cooking.

When the chicken is browned, remove it from the pan and set it aside on a plate. Turn the heat down to medium, and add the chicken broth and vinegar. Using a spatula, deglaze the pan, scraping up all the bits from the bottom of the pan. Add the garlic, onion, zucchini and tomatoes, and toss to coat them.

Add the chicken back to pan, nestling it in among the vegetables. Turn off the burner and using oven mitts, transfer the pan to the preheated oven. Bake uncovered for 45 minutes, or until the chicken is cooked through and the veggies are soft.

Serve as is or with a side of cauliflower rice or salad.

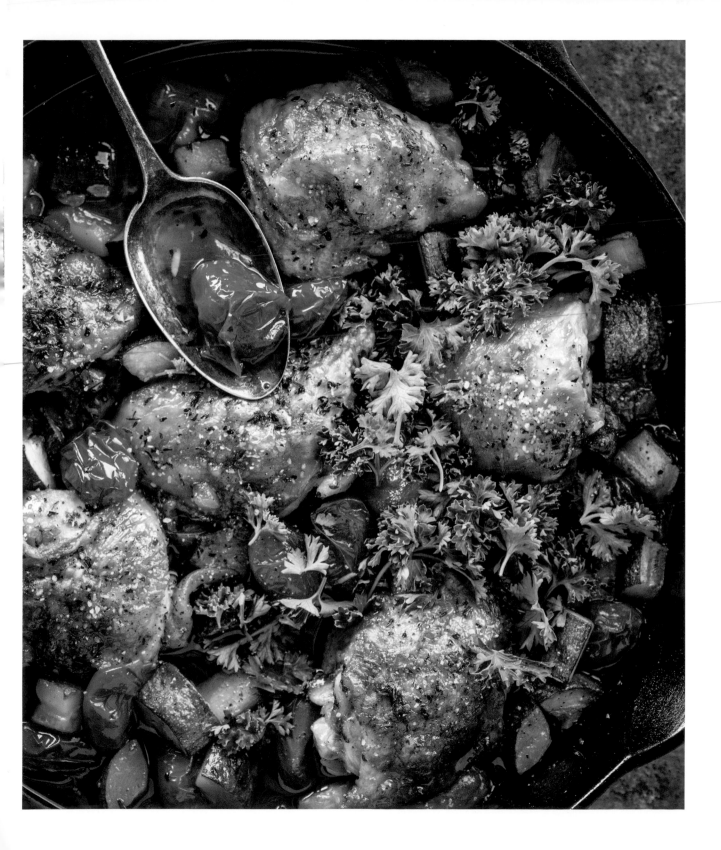

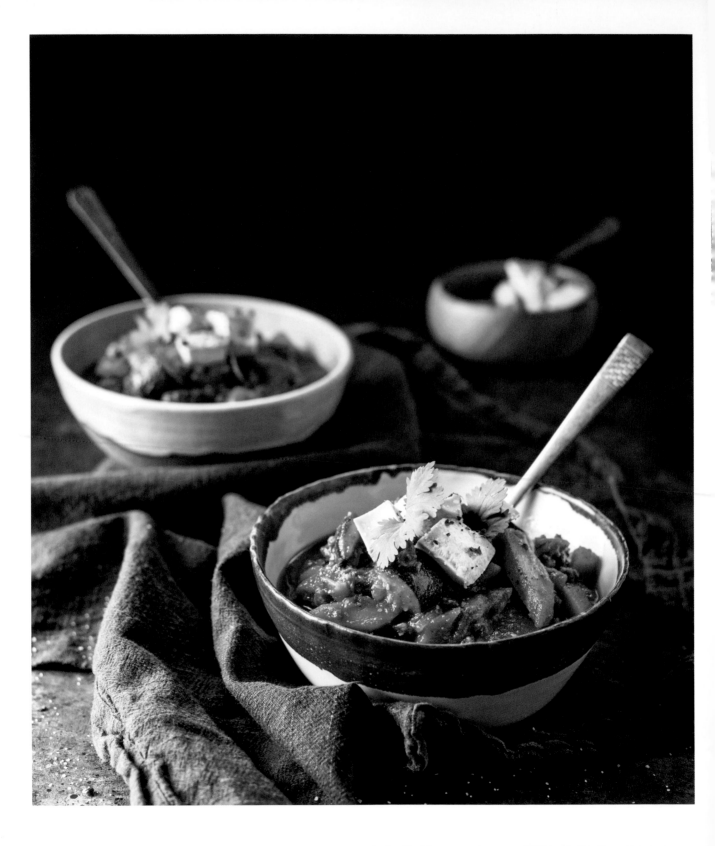

PALEO CHILI

Chili always makes me think of the fall. It's the perfect hearty and filling meal that warms you up when it's cold outside. I love serving this alongside my Grain-Free Almond Flour Bread (page 100). It's the perfect dipping companion!

SERVES 8

3 tbsp (45 ml) avocado oil, divided

1½ lb (680 g) ground beef

2 cloves garlic, chopped

1 large onion, diced

2 celery ribs, chopped

3 carrots, chopped

2 tbsp (15 g) chili powder

1 tsp ground cumin

1 tsp oregano

1 tsp salt

¼ tsp cayenne pepper (optional)

¼ tsp red pepper flakes (optional)

2 zucchini, diced

1 (15-oz [425-g]) can tomato puree or tomato sauce

1 (15-oz [425-g]) can diced tomatoes

Sliced avocado, for serving (optional)

Grain-Free Almond Flour Bread (page 100), for serving

Heat a Dutch oven over medium heat. Add 2 tablespoons (30 ml) of avocado oil, along with the ground beef and garlic. Cook over medium heat until the beef is thoroughly browned and no longer pink, about 15 minutes, making sure to break up and crumble the beef as you cook it. Drain off the excess fat and set the beef aside.

Add the remaining 1 tablespoon (15 ml) of oil, onion, celery, carrots, chili powder, cumin, oregano, salt, cayenne pepper (if using) and red pepper flakes (if using) to the Dutch oven. Cook the onion until it's translucent over medium-high heat, about 5 to 7 minutes. When the onion is golden and the veggies are midway cooked, add the zucchini and cook for 2 minutes, making sure you stir everything together well.

Add the cooked beef back to the Dutch oven. Add the tomato puree and diced tomatoes, and stir well. Turn the heat to high and bring everything to a boil, stirring frequently, then reduce the heat and simmer for 20 minutes. Every 5 minutes give the chili a good stir. Serve topped with avocado (if using) and a slice of grain-free bread.

NOTE: If you find the mixture is too thick, feel free to add 1 cup (240 ml) extra of tomato sauce or water.

CHICKEN AND TOMATO INSTANT POT STEW

This recipe is so full of flavor and quick to make when you're stuck in a time rut. You can serve it as is or over some Garlicky Cauliflower Rice (page 194). On its own it is quite filling and perfectly satiating. This recipe reminds me of my time spent in Italy. The olives, fresh herbs and tomatoes—oh the magic of Italy. Every time I eat a bowl of this stew, I'm reminded of the freshness of the food and the beautiful culture. I hope this recipe can mentally transport you there too!

SERVES 4

½ tbsp (5 g) sea salt, divided

8 boneless skinless chicken thighs

1 tbsp (15 ml) avocado or olive oil

1 onion, chopped

2 medium carrots, chopped

½ lb (226 g) cremini mushrooms, stems removed and cut into quarters

3 cloves garlic, chopped

1 tbsp (16 g) tomato paste

2 cups (298 g) cherry tomatoes

⅓ cup (45 g) sweet drop peppers, or to taste

½ cup (90 g) pitted green olives

2 tsp (3 g) dried basil

2 tsp (3 g) dried oregano

1 tsp red pepper flakes

¼ cup (15 g) loosely packed fresh Italian parsley, coarsely chopped

Cauliflower rice, for serving (optional)

Sprinkle ¾ teaspoon of sea salt onto your chicken thighs and set them aside. On your Instant Pot, press the Sauté button and then set to Medium Sauté. Add the avocado oil. When the oil is hot, add the onion, carrots, mushrooms and remaining sea salt. Sauté the vegetables until they have softened, about 3 to 5 minutes.

Add the garlic and tomato paste, and cook for about 30 seconds or until it's fragrant. Add the salted chicken, tomatoes, drop peppers, olives, basil, oregano, red pepper flakes and parsley to the pot. Stir everything together to combine.

Turn off the Sauté function, place the lid on your Instant Pot and set the vent in the lock position.

Press the Manual button, and set the cooking timer to 10 minutes. When cooking is complete, manually release the pressure. Serve as is or over cauliflower rice.

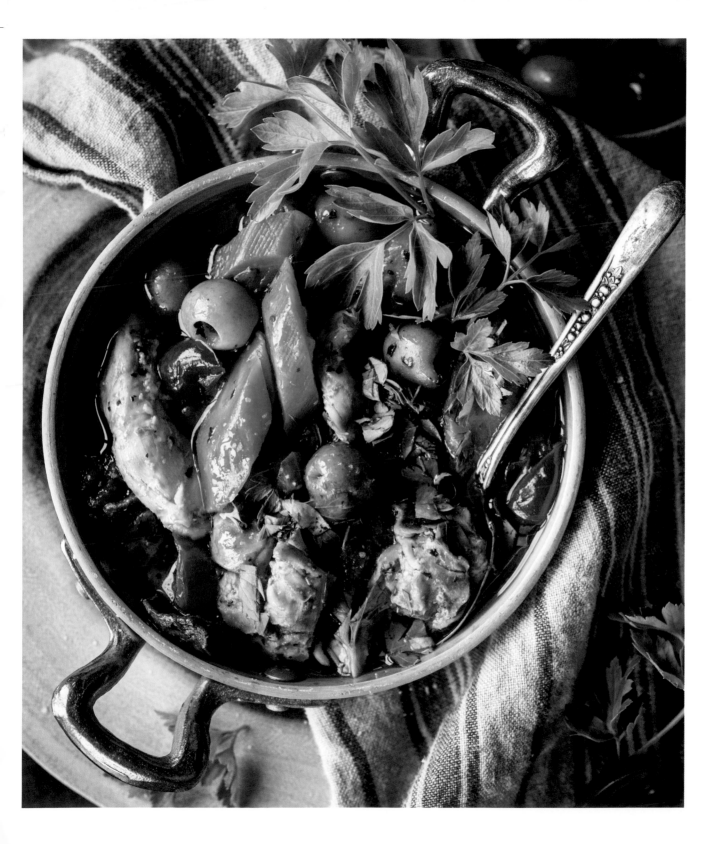

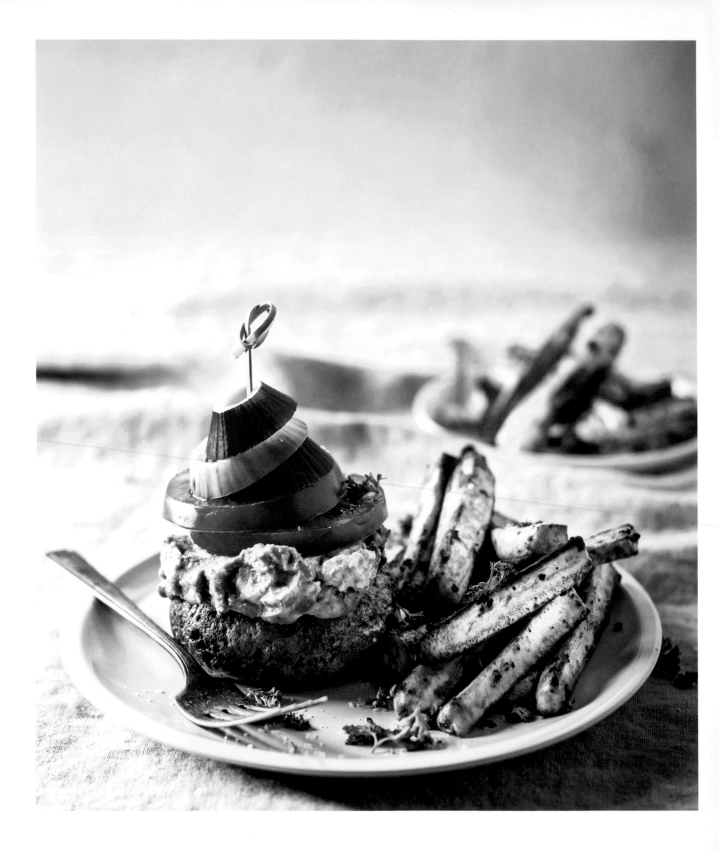

LAMB BURGERS WITH PLANTAIN FRIES

Lamb is a wonderful source of highly available iron, which can be helpful for those dealing with anemia. Of course, you can always use ground beef, chicken or turkey for this recipe—but when it comes to protein, variety is key. I like to spread on some Dijon mustard, BBQ sauce, one slice of tomato, a few slices of red onion and then finish it off with some guac. Served alongside plantain fries, this might just become your favorite weeknight meal. The spice mix for the plantain fries is AIP-approved (Autoimmune Paleo Protocol), and it is amazing on chicken or fish or roasted veggies. Use the guacamole recipe from the Paleo Taco Bowl (page 124) on your burger, and be sure to make extra for dipping your fries into!

SERVES 2 TO 3

FOR THE BURGERS

1 lb (454 g) ground lamb

2 tbsp (30 ml) coconut aminos

2 tsp (3 g) dried oregano

2 tsp (5 g) onion powder

2 tsp (5 g) garlic powder

1 tsp dried coriander

1 tsp smoked sweet paprika

1 tbsp (14 g) coconut oil

FOR THE PLANTAIN FRIES

2 large green plantains

2 tsp (5 g) onion powder

2 tsp (5 g) garlic powder

1 tsp dried coriander

1 tsp turmeric

½ tsp sea salt

FOR THE BURGER TOPPINGS

Sliced tomato

Sliced red onion

Guacamole (page 124)

BBQ sauce

Dijon mustard

Ketchup

Preheat the oven to 425°F (220°C, or gas mark 7), and cover a baking sheet with parchment paper.

To make the burgers, in a large bowl, add the lamb, coconut aminos, oregano, onion powder, garlic powder, coriander and sweet paprika. Use your hands to combine them. Divide the mixture into 3 equal parts and shape it into burger patties.

Heat a skillet over medium-high heat and add the coconut oil. Place the burgers in the skillet and cook for roughly 6 to 8 minutes on each side. Depending on the thickness of your burgers, you may need to cook them for more or less time on each side. Cook according to your preference. If you like them more well-done, cover the skillet with a lid, making sure to flip the burgers halfway through.

To make the plantain fries, prepare the plantains by cutting off both ends with a paring knife. Then cut the plantains in half down the middle. Run the paring knife down the length of each piece, making a cut deep enough to go through the skin but not into the flesh. Peel off the green skin and discard. Slice the plantains in half. You should end up with four halves. Slice each half into fries, and place the fries into a large bowl.

Mix the onion powder, garlic powder, coriander, turmeric and sea salt together in a small bowl. Add them to the plantains and thoroughly mix them together with your hands. Spread the fries out evenly onto a baking sheet and bake for 25 minutes, making sure to flip them halfway through the baking time.

Top your burger with your favorite toppings.

ROASTED TURKEY THIGHS

This is hands down my husband Gaetan's favorite recipe. There's just something about it that makes you feel like you're enjoying a lavish Thanksgiving dinner without all the hoopla! I find it challenging to get turkey thighs year-round, but right around Thanksgiving and Christmas I make sure to stock up and freeze a few. This recipe is ideal for those who love dark meat—that's me! Serve this alongside some Garlicky Cauliflower Rice (page 194) and Roasted Asparagus (page 190) for the perfect dinner.

SERVES 4

4 (1-lb [454-g]) bone-in, skin-on turkey thighs

⅓ cup (75 g) butter

5–6 fresh sage leaves, roughly chopped

2 cloves garlic, roughly chopped

1 tsp sea salt

Preheat the oven to 375°F (190°C, or gas mark 5), and line a baking sheet with parchment paper. Place the turkey thighs on the baking sheet.

In a pot over medium heat, melt the butter together with the sage, garlic and sea salt. Keep it on a low heat for 5 to 6 minutes, letting the sage and garlic infuse the butter. Remove the butter from the heat and pour it evenly over all four thighs. Use your hands to rub it all over the turkey, making sure to rub the mixture into the meat, under the skin.

Roast the thighs for 40 to 50 minutes, or until a meat thermometer registers 170°F (77°C).

Turn the oven to a low broil and broil for 5 to 7 minutes, until the skin on the top gets crispy. Be sure to watch the thighs as some ovens broil faster than others and you want to avoid burning the skin.

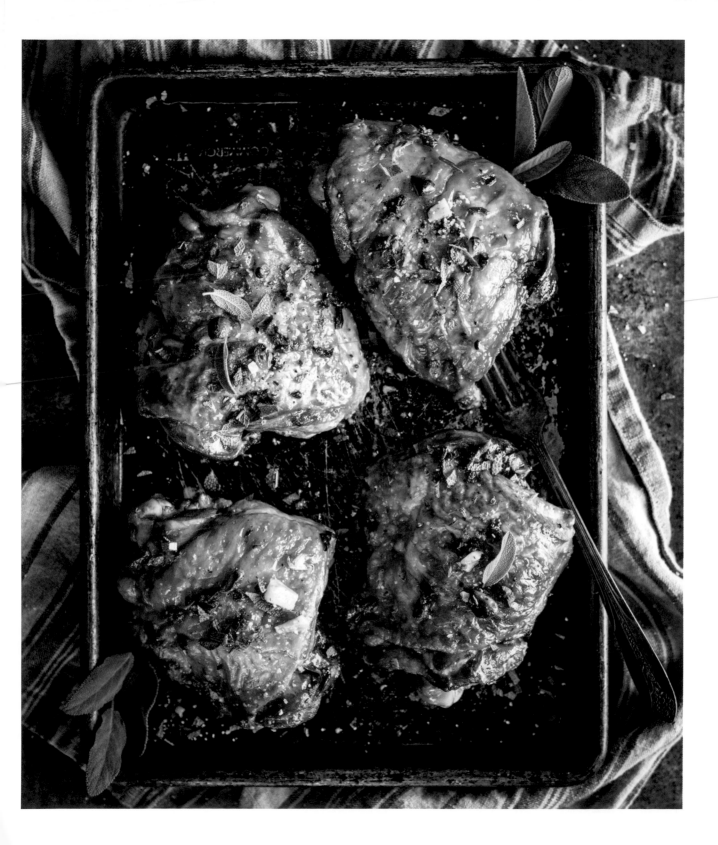

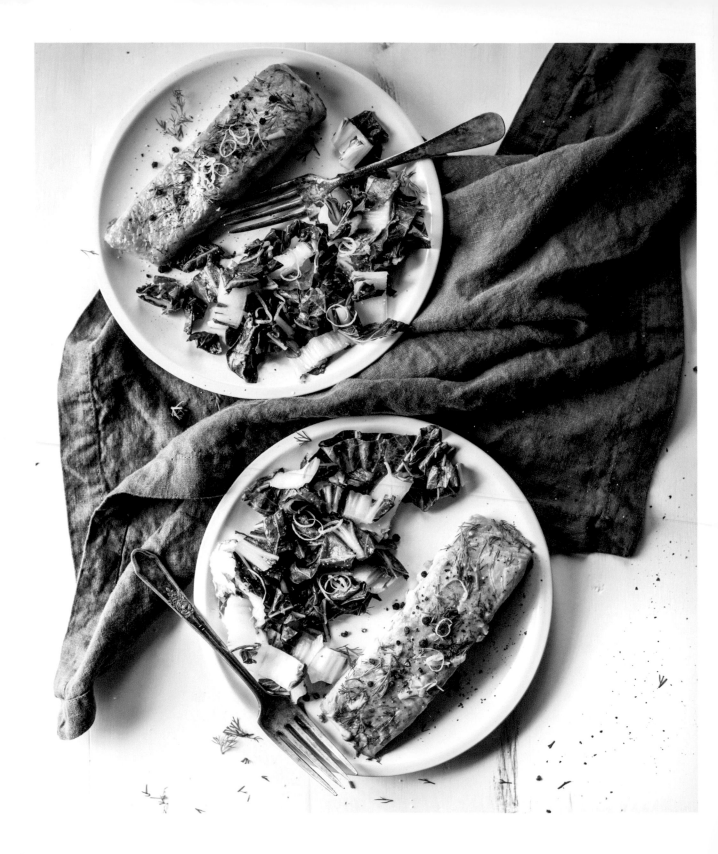

DIJON-DILL HERBED WILD SALMON

My mother is Portuguese, so growing up we ate a lot of fish. It's important to choose wild fish over farmed to avoid PCBs (polychlorinated biphenyls) or antibiotics. Although wild fish may have a higher price tag, it's definitely worth the purchase. Quality is so important when sourcing fish, especially with the high amount of contaminates and toxins lurking in our ocean. I love wild salmon for the incredible omega-3 content which has anti-inflammatory benefits. I like to serve this salmon alongside some wilted greens for an easy weeknight dinner.

SERVES 2

2 (6-oz [170-g]) portions of wild salmon

2 tbsp (30 ml) Dijon mustard

1 tbsp (15 ml) olive oil

2 tsp (3 g) chopped fresh dill

Juice of 1 lemon

2 cloves garlic, chopped

Pinch of sea salt and pepper

Preheat the oven to 350°F (175°C, or gas mark 4), and line a baking sheet with parchment paper. Place the salmon on the baking sheet.

In a bowl, whisk together the Dijon mustard, olive oil, dill, lemon juice, garlic, sea salt and pepper. Spread the mixture onto the salmon. Bake for 15 minutes, or until the salmon is pink and flaky.

BAKED SEA BASS WITH PINEAPPLE SALSA

Sea bass is often referred to as the "steak of fish." It's buttery and creamy, and it happens to be my absolute favorite! Combined with the freshness of the pineapple salsa, it's a match made in heaven. I often look for Chilean sea bass at my local fish market, and I buy a few extra when it's on sale. If you're not a fish fan, sea bass has a very mild taste and the texture is often a fan favorite—so give it a try. Serve this alongside some Roasted Asparagus (page 190), a simple salad or Broccoli Rice (page 197) for a delicious heart-healthy meal.

SERVES 1

FOR THE SEA BASS

1 (6-oz [170-g]) sea bass fillet

Sea salt and black pepper

½ tbsp (8 ml) melted grass-fed butter

FOR THE PINEAPPLE SALSA

½ cup (83 g) fresh chopped pineapple

1 tbsp (10 g) chopped red onion

1 tbsp (1 g) cilantro, chopped

1 clove garlic, chopped

1 tsp apple cider vinegar

⅛ tsp cayenne pepper, or to taste (optional)

Sea salt and black pepper

To make the sea bass, preheat the oven to 425°F (220°C, or gas mark 7). Line a baking sheet with parchment paper.

Lightly sprinkle the fish with sea salt and pepper, drizzle it with the melted butter and place it on the prepared baking sheet. Bake in the oven for 12 to 16 minutes, or until the fish is cooked through. Depending on the thickness of your fish, it may take a little longer.

To make the salsa, while the fish is cooking, mix together the pineapple, onion, cilantro, garlic, vinegar and cayenne, if using, together in a bowl. Season with sea salt and pepper to taste, and set it aside.

Remove the fish from the oven, and serve with pineapple salsa over the top.

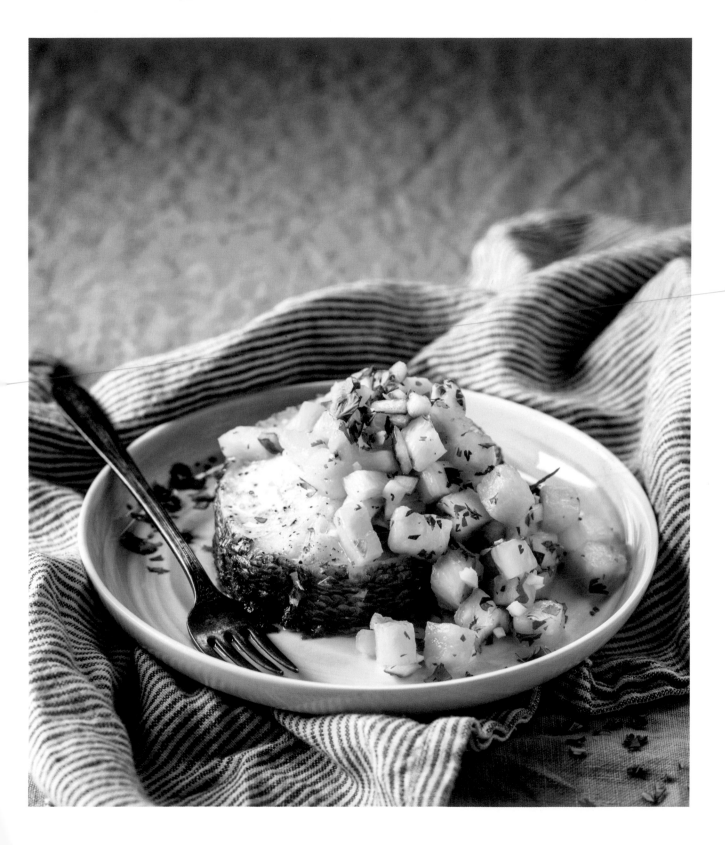

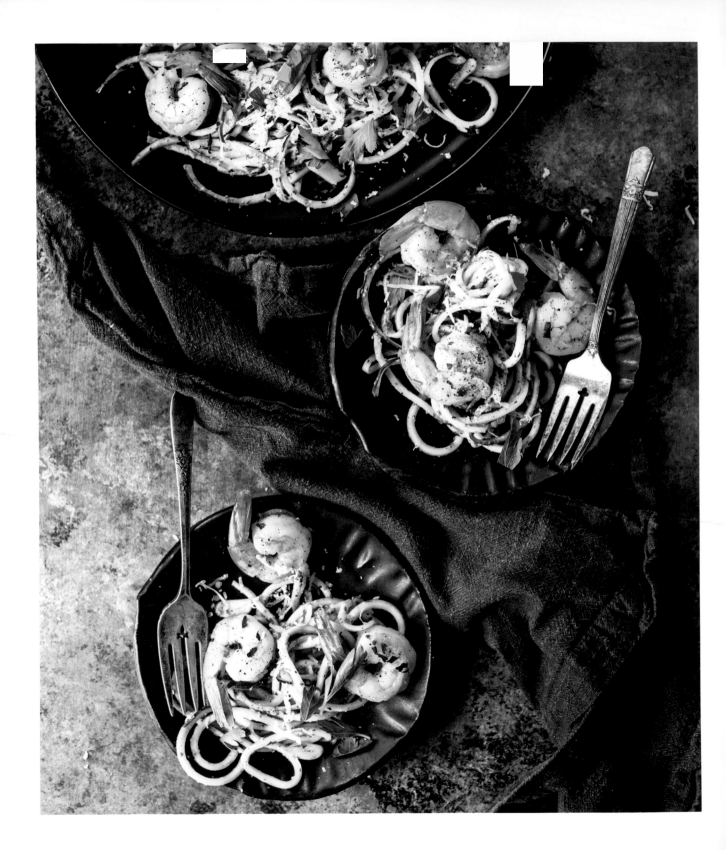

GARLIC SHRIMP WITH WALNUT PESTO ZOODLES

Cooking up a meal for a family of four doesn't need to be time consuming. This recipe is perfect when you need a quick and healthy meal. Shrimp is a great source of protein, plus it provides a healthy dose of selenium, zinc and iron. Combine it with some pesto zoodles and you have a ten-minute meal that is hearty and delicious.

SERVES 4

FOR THE WALNUT PESTO (OPTIONAL)

1 cup (117 g) raw walnuts or pine nuts

3 cups (72 g) fresh basil leaves

2 cups (60 g) fresh baby spinach leaves

4 cloves garlic

⅔ cup (160 ml) olive oil

¾ tsp sea salt

2 tbsp (16 g) nutritional yeast or Parmesan cheese (if you can tolerate dairy)

FOR THE SHRIMP AND ZOODLES

2 large zucchini

3 tbsp (45 ml) olive oil, for sautéing

1 large bag frozen shrimp, defrosted and shells off (roughly 30–40 shrimp)

3 cloves garlic, chopped

1 tsp red pepper flakes, or more to taste

2 tbsp (4 g) roughly chopped fresh parsley

Sea salt and black pepper

¼ cup (60 g) Walnut Pesto or store-bought

To make the walnut pesto (if using), place the walnuts, basil, spinach, garlic, olive oil, sea salt and nutritional yeast into a food processor. Blend until they're well combined and set it aside. You will have more pesto than what is needed for the recipe. Store the extra in a mason jar in the fridge for up to 1 week, and use it with chicken or fish or as a veggie dip.

Spiralize the zucchini and set it aside. I like to use the ¼-inch (6-mm) blade on my spiralizer for a thicker noodle.

Heat a cast-iron skillet over medium heat. Add the olive oil. When it's hot, add the shrimp, garlic, red pepper flakes, parsley, sea salt and black pepper to taste.

Cook for 2 to 3 minutes on each side, until the shrimp is cooked through and nicely pink. Remove the shrimp from the skillet and place them in a bowl.

To the same skillet, add the zucchini noodles and pesto. Cook for roughly 5 to 7 minutes over medium heat, until the desired texture is reached and the zucchini is slightly softened.

Add the zoodles to a bowl and top with the shrimp.

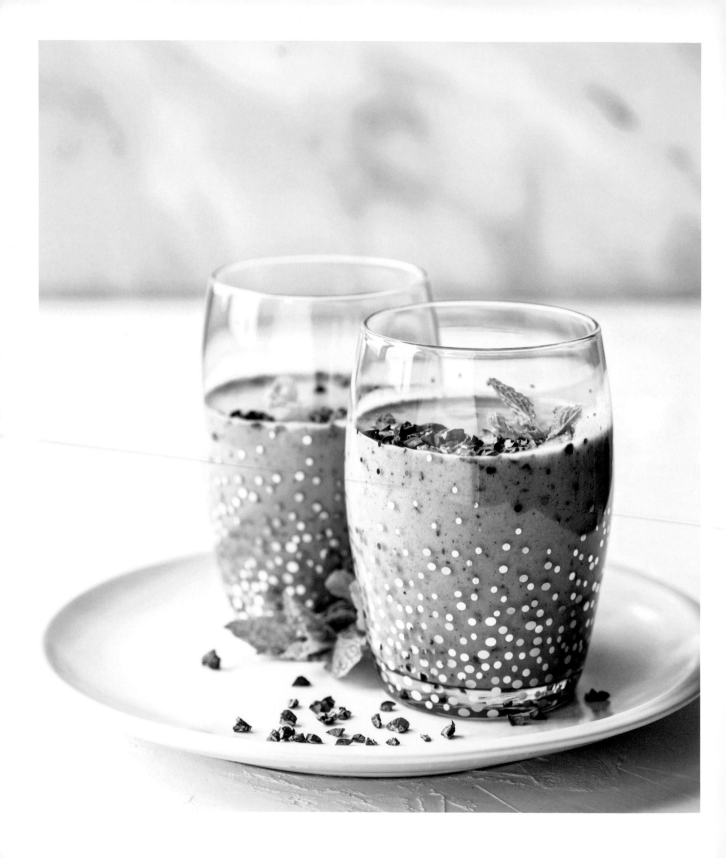

SMOOTHIES AND ELIXIRS

MINT CHOCOLATE CHIP SMOOTHIE

The combination of mint and chocolate is my absolute favorite. I remember as a kid going to Baskin-Robbins, I always ordered the mint chocolate ice cream. Nowadays, regular ice cream and I do not go well together. Enter this smoothie. This is the perfect balance of protein, fat and fiber, with just the right amount of sweetness. You'll think you're having dessert for breakfast. But no, it's just simple whole foods that taste delicious and support your hormones.

SERVES 1

1 small frozen banana

2 cups (480 ml) unsweetened coconut milk

1 cup (30 g) fresh spinach

¼ small/medium avocado

10–20 fresh mint leaves OR 1 drop peppermint essential oil

1 scoop vanilla or chocolate protein powder or collagen peptides (chocolate could change the color of your smoothie, but who cares—it'll still be delish)

½ cup (120 g) crushed ice, or more if you like it thicker

1 tbsp (20 g) cacao nibs or chocolate chips, plus more for garnish

Place the banana, coconut milk, spinach, avocado, mint, protein powder and ice in a blender. Process until it's smooth. Add the cacao nibs and briefly pulse. Serve garnished with additional cacao nibs and enjoy!

CHOCOLATE CHERRY BOMB SMOOTHIE

I think there was probably a span of 60 days where all I had for breakfast was this smoothie—true story. It's so creamy and delicious, and the ingredients are hormone-balancing perfection. The frozen cauliflower offers up amazing fiber, plus sulforaphane, which helps the liver detox excess estrogen. The ground flaxseeds also help to support estrogen detox by binding to excess estrogen in the gut and flushing it out through the bowels. This is one gut-loving, liver detox–friendly smoothie that tastes incredible.

SERVES 1

2 cups (480 ml) almond or coconut milk

2 scoops chocolate protein powder

⅓ cup (51 g) frozen cherries

⅓ cup (33 g) frozen cauliflower

1 tbsp (16 g) almond or sunflower seed butter

1 tbsp (10 g) flaxseeds, freshly ground

Add the almond milk, protein powder, cherries, cauliflower, almond butter and flaxseeds to a high-speed blender. Blend on high until they're well combined.

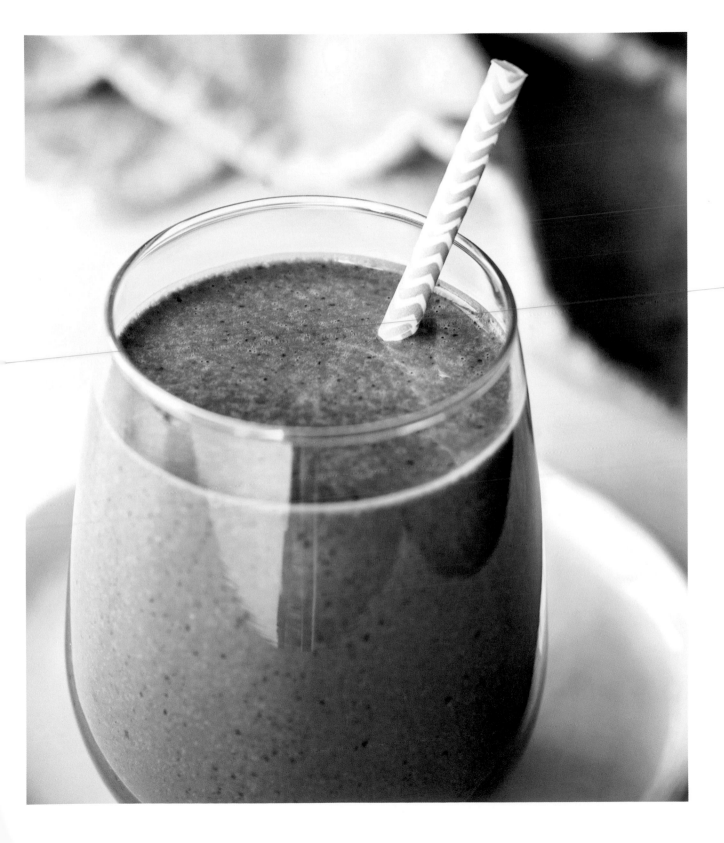

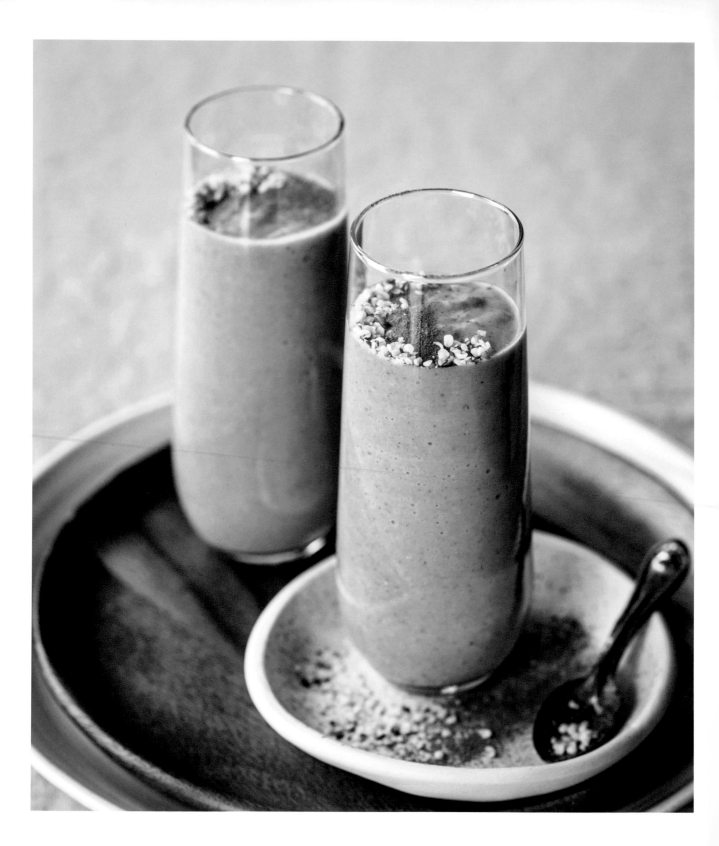

PUMPKIN PIE SMOOTHIE

I absolutely love pumpkin. Knowing that I can pick up organic canned pumpkin puree any time of year makes me so happy. Adding pumpkin to your smoothies is a great way to get in additional fiber, low-glycemic carbs and antioxidants. Be sure to pick up pumpkin puree and not pumpkin pie mix.

SERVES 1

2 cups (480 ml) almond or coconut milk

⅓ cup (81 g) pumpkin puree

½ frozen banana

1 scoop vanilla protein powder

1 tbsp (16 g) almond or cashew butter

1 tbsp (7 g) hemp seeds, plus extra for sprinkling

1 tsp ground cinnamon

1 tsp pumpkin pie spice

Add the almond milk, pumpkin, banana, protein powder, almond butter, hemp seeds, cinnamon and pumpkin pie spice to a blender. Blend on high until they're well combined. Sprinkle with hemp seeds to garnish.

SWEET GREENS SMOOTHIE

My green smoothies are so near and dear to me. It's easy to throw a few handfuls of greens into your blender and instantly feel the energizing and alkalizing benefits. Kale and spinach can be quite bitter when eaten raw. Combining them with sweet pineapple gives this smoothie the perfect sweetness, plus it feels like you're drinking a healthy piña colada!

Pineapple contains bromelain, an enzyme that helps aid in digestion. If you need more digestive support, feel free to add a capsule of your favorite probiotic. Simply open the capsule and pour in the powder. Once you mix it up, you'll never know it's in there.

SERVES 1

2 cups (480 ml) coconut milk

½ cup (83 g) fresh chopped pineapple

Large handful of kale, de-stemmed

Large handful of spinach

1 tbsp (7 g) hemp seeds, plus extra for sprinkling

1 tsp chia seeds, plus extra for sprinkling

1 scoop vanilla protein powder

1 tsp ground cinnamon

1 probiotic capsule (optional)

Add the coconut milk, pineapple, kale, spinach, hemp seeds, chia seeds, protein powder, cinnamon and probiotic, if using, to a blender. Blend on high until they're well combined. Sprinkle with hemp and chia seeds to garnish.

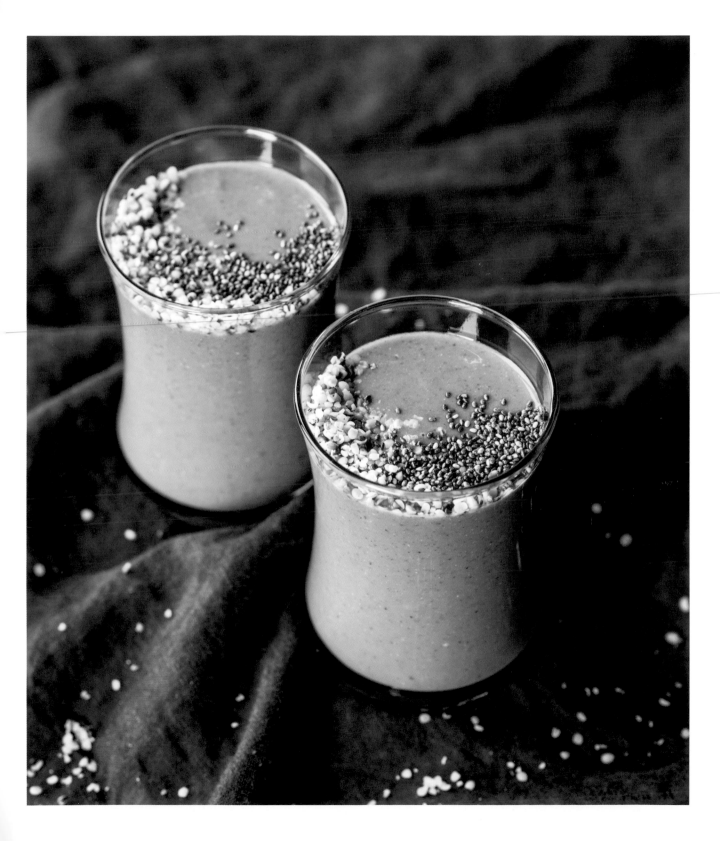

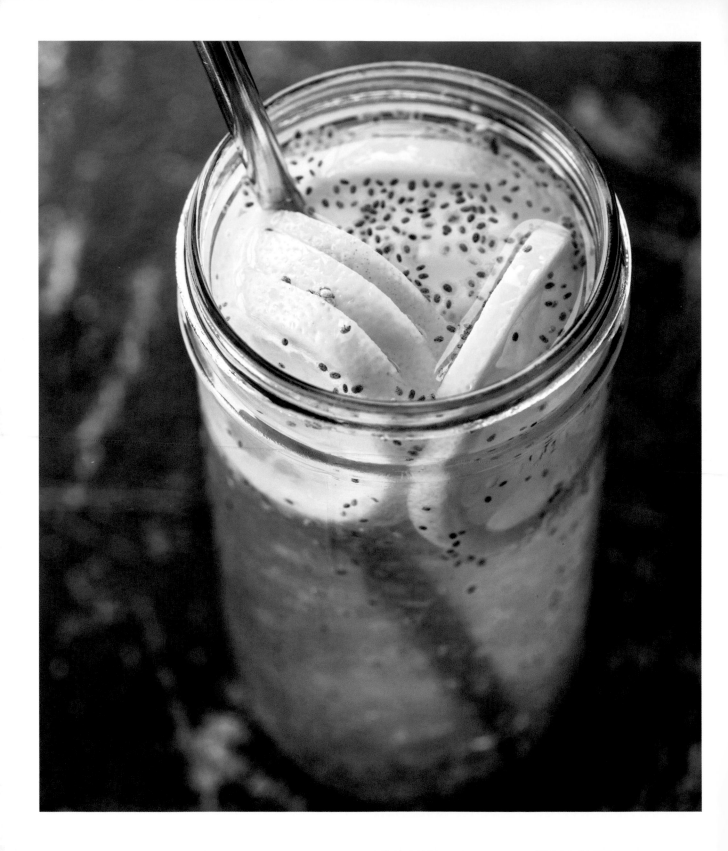

CHIA LEMON PRE-WORKOUT SHAKE

Chia seeds are an amazing way to retain electrolytes and fuel your body for a workout. This shake is great as a pre-workout drink—or even during a workout to maintain electrolyte balance. I love these incredible seeds for many reasons—protein, fat and fiber. It's really a winning combination. This shake contains no artificial sweeteners or chemical additives; most pre-workout sports drinks do. Natural is the way to go!

SERVES 1

2 cups (480 ml) springwater

1–2 tsp (3–6 g) chia seeds

Juice of ½ lemon

½ tsp raw honey or maple syrup (optional)

Lemon slices, for garnish

Add the water, chia seeds, lemon juice and honey, if using, to a shaker cup or mason jar. Shake well. Garnish with lemon slices. Enjoy before your workout or sip during exercise.

POST-WORKOUT RECOVERY SHAKE

This shake is perfectly refreshing right after a workout, and it is loaded with whole food electrolytes. Plus, it contains just enough sugar to help replace glycogen stores after your intense workout. It's time to ditch the high-sugar and calorie-dense artificial recovery shakes. Start making your own using the natural sweetness from real food.

SERVES 1

2 cups (480 ml) coconut water

Juice of 1 lemon

Juice of 1 lime

1 Medjool date, pitted

2 tsp (10 g) camu camu powder

1 scoop collagen powder or your favorite protein powder

½ tsp sea salt

Add the coconut water, lemon juice, lime juice, date, camu camu, collagen powder and sea salt to a blender. Blend on high until they're well combined.

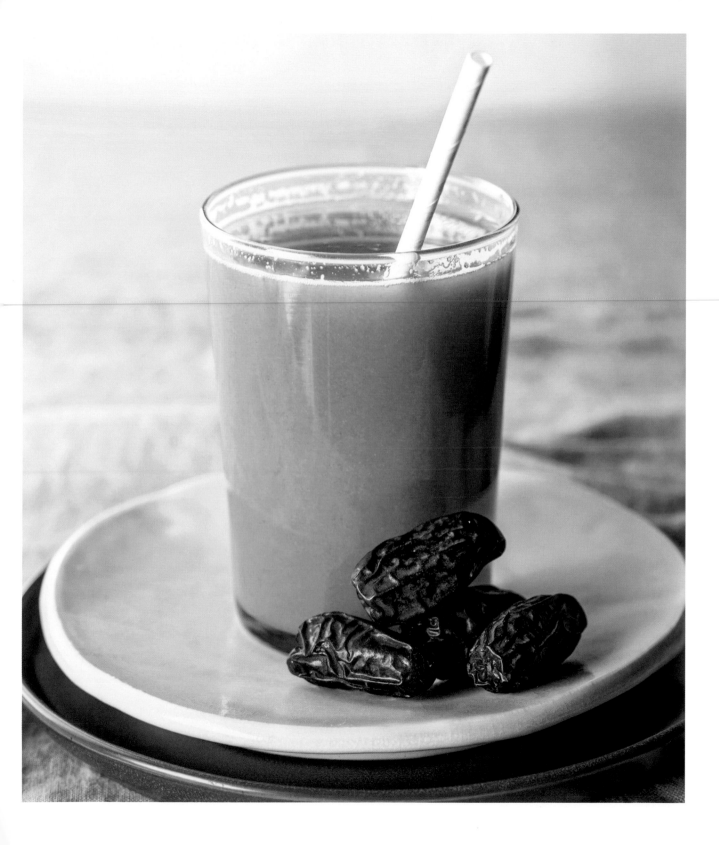

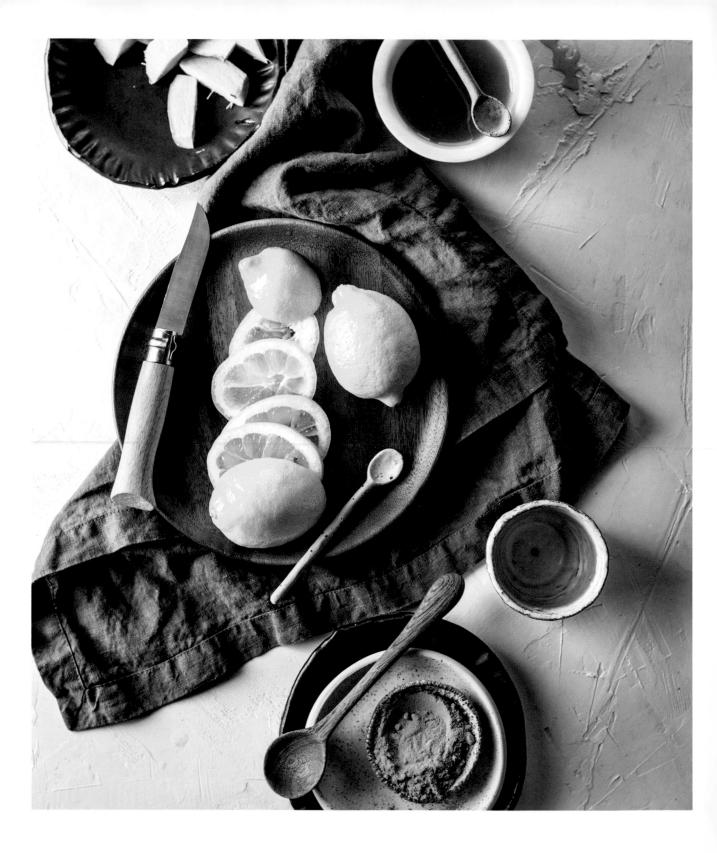

GINGER TURMERIC LEMONADE

This lemonade can be enjoyed hot during the winter months and cool in the summer. It's so versatile and incredibly healing. Ginger is a natural anti-inflammatory and helps to fire up your digestive juices, making it easier for you to digest your food and nutrients. Turmeric helps to support the liver by protecting it against toxic damage, and lemon helps to purify the blood and protect your immune system due to its high vitamin C content.

SERVES 4

4 cups (960 ml) springwater, plus more if needed

3- to 4-inch (7.5- to 10-cm) piece of fresh organic ginger

1 tsp organic turmeric powder

Juice of 2 organic lemons

1 tsp raw honey (optional)

Add the water and ginger to a pot. Simmer on the stove over medium-low heat for about 20 minutes.

If enjoying the drink hot, strain it into a mug. Add the turmeric, lemon juice and honey (if using), and stir. Keep the remaining water and ginger in a pot on the stove, and reheat for later use.

If enjoying it cold, strain it into a large mason jar. Add in the turmeric, lemon juice and honey (if using). Top it up with 4 to 5 cups (960 ml to 1.2 L) of room-temperature water. Place it in the fridge until it's chilled, 3 to 4 hours, for a cold lemonade.

ANTI-INFLAMMATORY TURMERIC LATTE

Collagen is a superfood that has gotten a ton of buzz in the last few years—and for good reason. From beautifying your skin to supporting your joints to healing your gut, it truly is a healing superfood. I love combining it with anti-inflammatory turmeric in this delicious elixir.

SERVES 1

2 cups (480 ml) unsweetened coconut milk

1 tbsp (6 g) collagen powder

1 tbsp (7 g) hemp seeds

½ tbsp (3 g) turmeric powder, or more to taste

1 tsp ground cinnamon, plus more for sprinkling

1 tsp ground ginger

Pinch of sea salt

Your choice of sweetener (raw honey, maple syrup or monk fruit)

Heat the coconut milk in a pot on the stovetop over medium heat. When it's hot, add the milk to your blender with the collagen powder, hemp seeds, turmeric, cinnamon, ginger, sea salt and sweetener. Blend on high until they're well combined. Sprinkle with cinnamon to garnish.

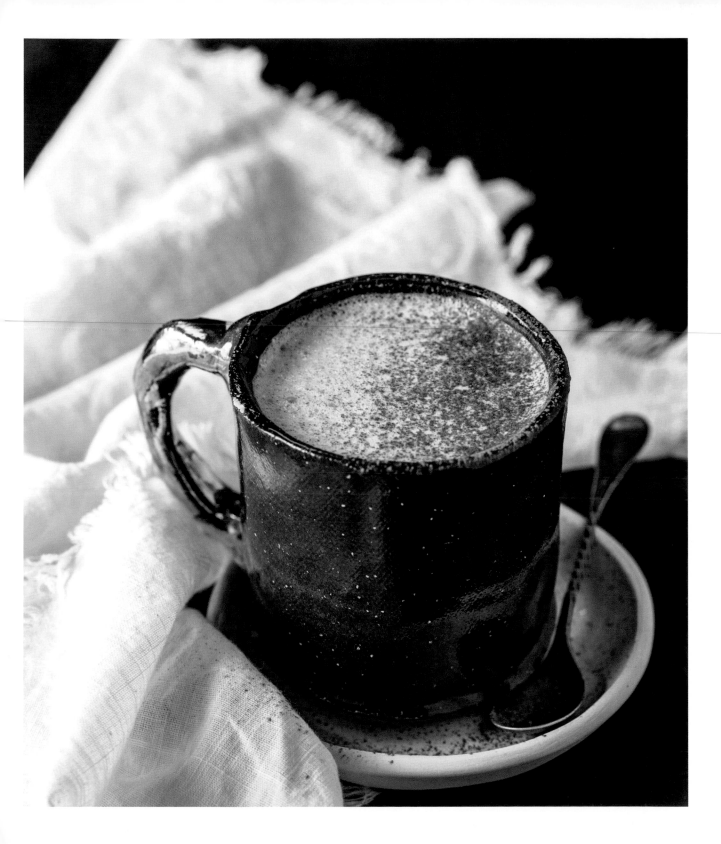

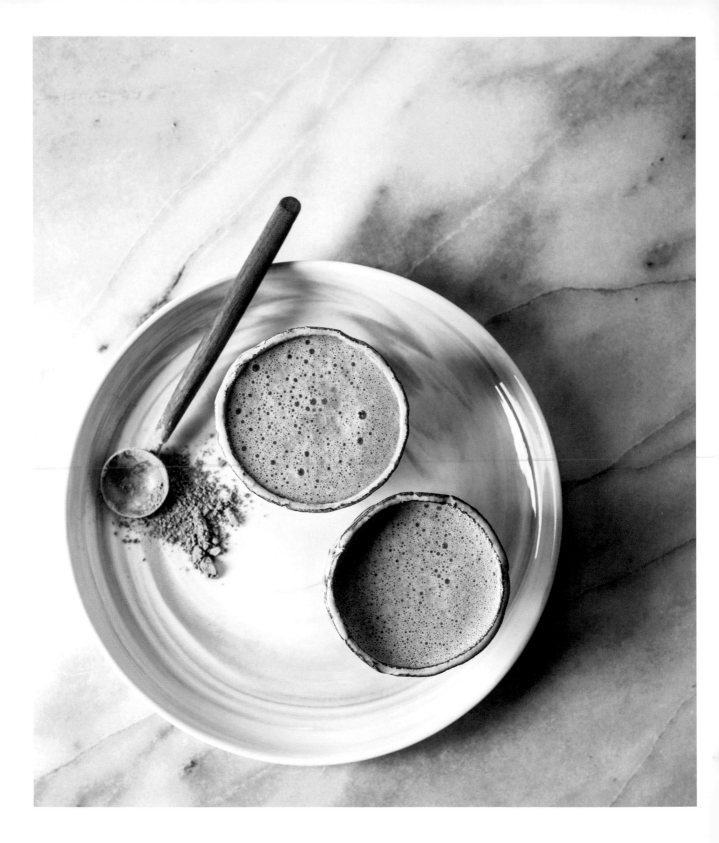

MATCHA GREEN TEA LATTE

If you're looking for an alternative to your daily coffee, matcha is your best option! It's loaded with antioxidants and offers up a healthy dose of caffeine—not as much as your usual cup of java, but still enough to help give you that boost and support mental clarity.

SERVES 1

1½ cups (360 ml) unsweetened coconut milk or nut milk

1 tbsp (6 g) collagen powder

1 tbsp (6 g) matcha powder

1 tsp ground cinnamon

1 tsp raw honey or sweetener of choice

Heat the coconut milk in a pot on the stovetop over medium heat. When it's hot, add the milk to your blender with the collagen powder, matcha powder, cinnamon and honey. Blend on high until they're well combined.

COCONUT COLLAGEN COFFEE

This is my absolute favorite way to enjoy my morning coffee. Now, I'm all for a delicious and simple americano, but the combination of coconut butter and collagen gives this latte so much creaminess that I have a hard time going without it. Maybe this will become your new favorite way to enjoy your coffee too!

SERVES 1

1 cup (240 ml) fresh brewed hot coffee or americano or espresso

Hot water, add enough according to your preference

1 tbsp (6 g) collagen powder

½ tbsp (7 g) coconut butter

Brew your coffee according to your preference. I often make an americano, or I use 1 packet of Four Sigmatic coffee and add roughly 1 cup (240 ml) of hot boiling water.

Add the coffee to a blender with the collagen powder and coconut butter. Blend on high until they're well combined.

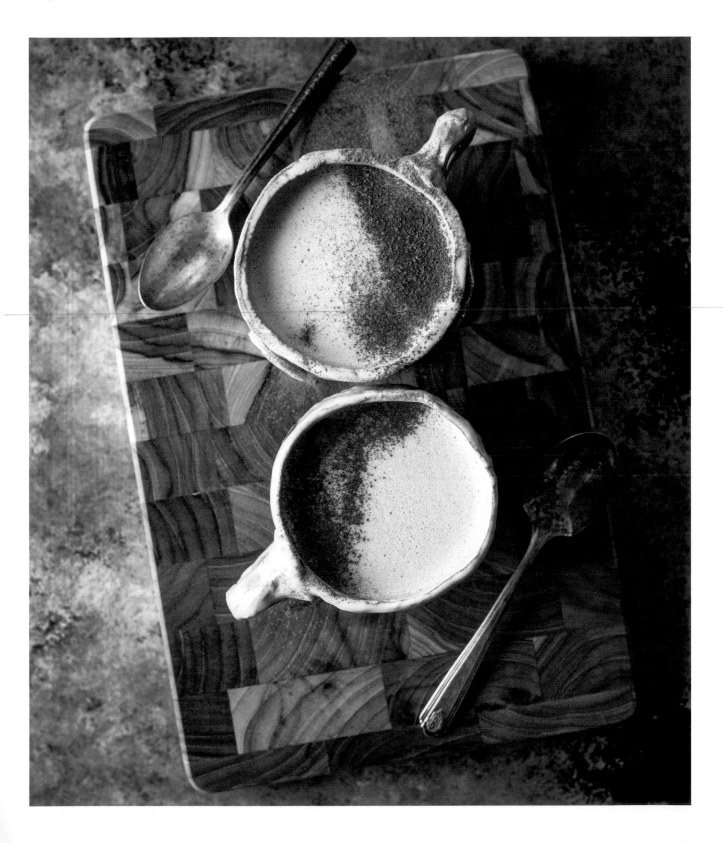

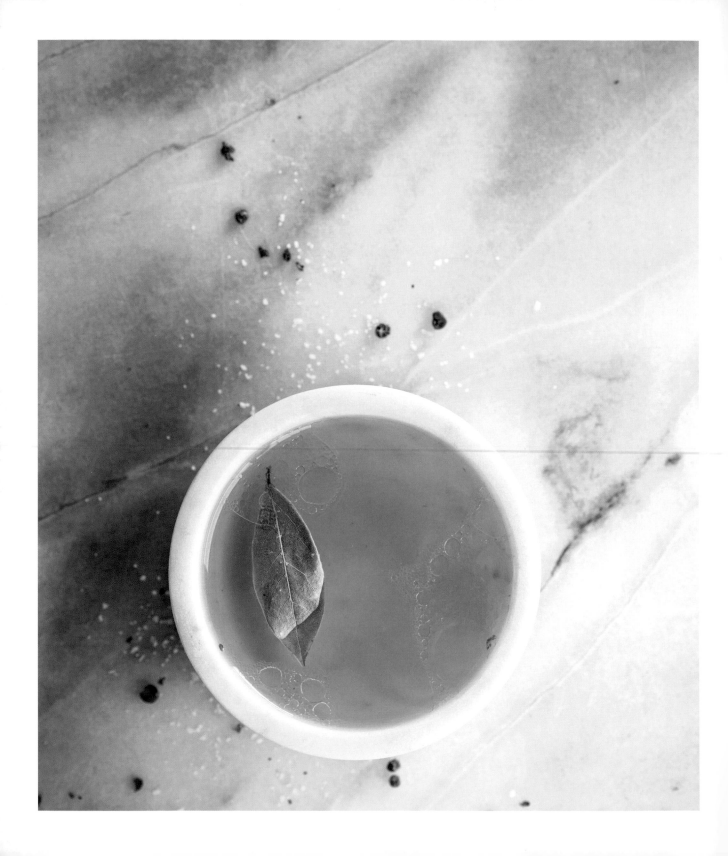

SOUPS AND SALADS

INSTANT POT CHICKEN BONE BROTH

This recipe is liquid gold right here. It's full of amino acids that help to heal the gut, and it is wonderful for skin and joint health, too. If you've been dealing with a ton of digestive or gut issues, or even autoimmune flare-ups, I highly recommend starting your day with a cup of warm bone broth. It's nourishing, delicious and incredibly simple to make. I make this recipe in my 6-quart (6-L) Instant Pot.

MAKES 14 TO 16 CUPS (3.4 TO 3.8 L)

1 leek, washed well and roughly chopped

2 celery ribs, roughly chopped

2 carrots, roughly chopped

1 onion, roughly chopped

5 cloves garlic, roughly chopped

4 or 5 sprigs of fresh thyme

1 bay leaf

5 or 6 chicken feet, or more depending on how big your pot is

1 lb (454 g) chicken wings or backs, or more depending on how big your pot is

1 tbsp (15 ml) gluten-free fish sauce

Add the leek, celery, carrots, onion, garlic, thyme, bay leaf and chicken to your Instant Pot.

Add filtered water to the fill line, and add the fish sauce. Give everything a good stir.

Select Manual on your Instant Pot, and set the timer for 150 minutes. Make sure the pressure valve is in the locked position. Wait for ON to appear—and you're all set.

When the timer is complete, release the pressure valve. Let the broth cool down for 30 minutes before straining it. I like to strain mine into mason jars, leaving them to cool completely in the fridge overnight before transferring them to the freezer. Only transfer the broth to the freezer if you won't be using it right away.

NOTE: I suggest you roughly chop up the chicken wings or backs to release more nutrients and gelatin. Ask your butcher to do it for you.

HEALING CHICKEN SOUP

There's nothing like whipping up a delicious chicken soup with your homemade broth. We've coined Sundays in our house as "bone broth Sundays." We make broth, then make soup and enjoy it for dinner with a light salad. The soup is gut healing and incredibly nourishing, and it's full of incredible healing vitamins, minerals and antioxidants. I hope it becomes your Sunday staple, too.

SERVES 6

3 lb (1.4 kg) boneless, skinless chicken thighs (fresh, not frozen)

6 cups (1.4 L) Instant Pot Chicken Bone Broth (page 165)

3 tbsp (18 g) grass-fed unflavored gelatin powder

1 yellow onion, chopped

5 cloves garlic, minced

2 tsp (4 g) ground turmeric

1 tbsp (9 g) sea salt, plus more to taste

2 celery ribs, chopped

2 carrots, chopped

1 sweet potato, chopped into 1-inch (2.5-cm) pieces

¼ cup (15 g) fresh flat-leaf parsley, roughly chopped

1½ tsp (1 g) fresh thyme leaves

1 bay leaf

2–3 tsp (10–15 ml) lemon juice (optional)

Place the chicken thighs in your Instant Pot. Add the bone broth, gelatin powder, onion, garlic, turmeric and sea salt. Secure the lid, set your pressure valve and select the Manual setting. Set to high pressure for 10 minutes.

When the 10 minutes is up, quick-release the pressure. Remove the chicken and cut it into 1-inch (2.5-cm) chunks. Return it to the Instant Pot.

Add the celery, carrots, sweet potato, parsley, thyme and bay leaf. Secure the lid again, set the pressure valve, select the Manual setting and set it to high pressure for 3 minutes. When the 3 minutes is up, quick-release the pressure.

Remove the bay leaf. Ladle the soup into bowls, and serve hot with lemon juice, if using.

NOTE: Feel free to stir in 2 cups (60 g) of fresh spinach at the very end. It's a great way to get in extra vitamin C.

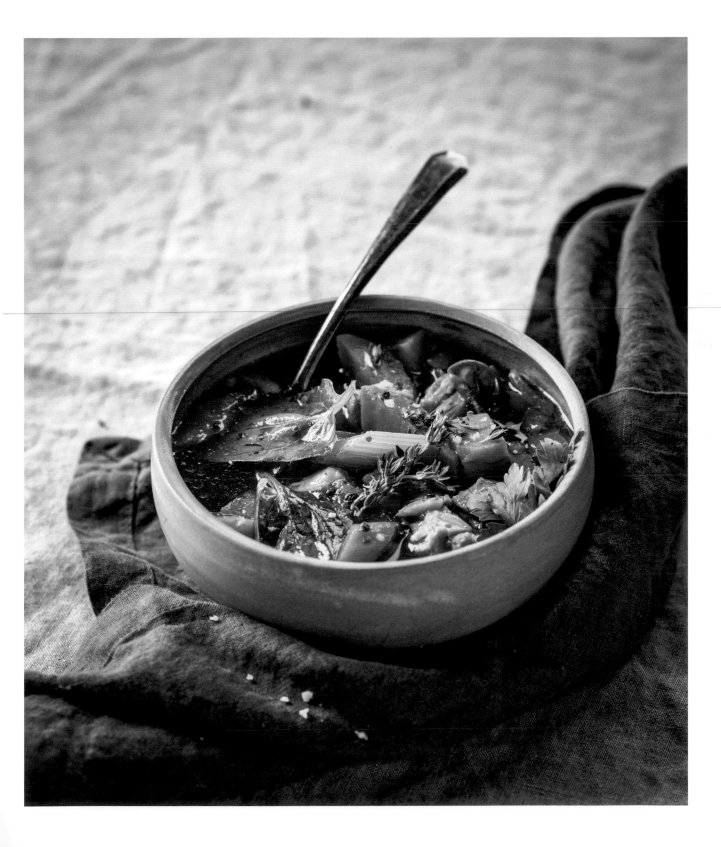

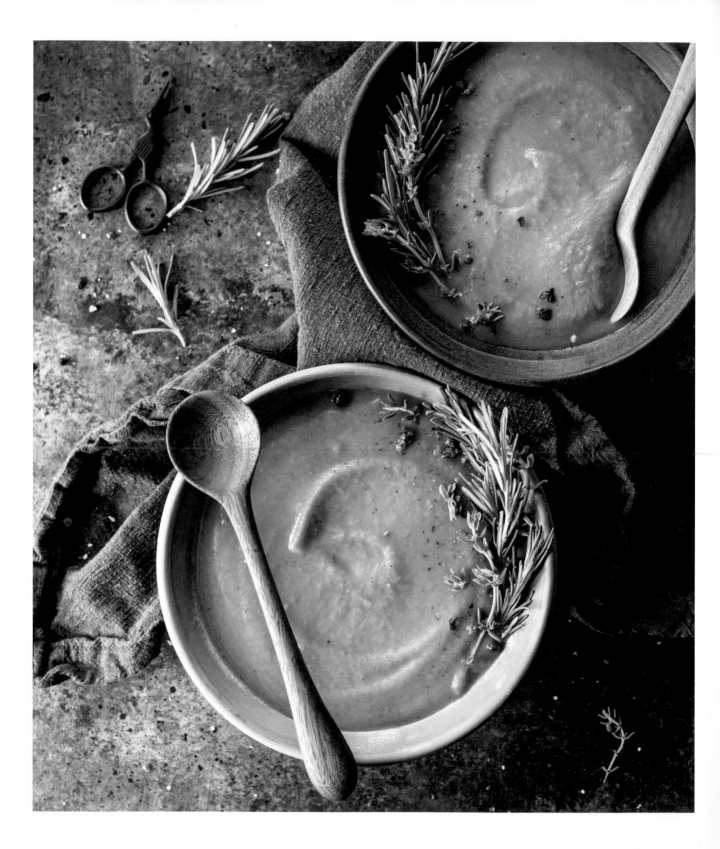

SWEET POTATO SOUP

Sweet potatoes are truly one of my favorite vegetables. They are incredibly versatile—from mashing them to making fries to enjoying them sweet or savory. They also contain a healthy dose of fiber, iron, beta-carotene and vitamin C.

SERVES 4

2 tbsp (30 ml) olive oil

1 onion, chopped

2 carrots, peeled and chopped

2 celery ribs, chopped

1 large sweet potato, cut into small 1-inch (2.5-cm) chunks

3 cups (720 ml) chicken broth

1 tbsp (8 g) ground cinnamon

½ tsp sea salt, or more to taste

Place a large pot over medium heat. Add the olive oil. When it begins to get hot, add the onion, carrots and celery. Sauté until the vegetables are softened, about 3 to 4 minutes.

Add the sweet potato and enough broth to completely cover all the vegetables. If you don't have enough broth, use water. Season with cinnamon and sea salt, and bring it to a simmer. Cook until the sweet potatoes are very soft, about 15 minutes, then puree the soup with a hand blender or transfer to a blender to puree. Taste and add more seasoning if necessary.

THE BIELER BROTH

This incredible broth is a gentle yet powerful way to help detox your body and improve your digestive track. It was created by Dr. Henry Bieler, a visionary American physician and author of *Food Is Your Best Medicine*. This broth is rich in potassium and sodium, alkalizes the body and supports the liver and the adrenal glands. It also helps the pancreas control blood sugar, which is key for women who are struggling with insulin resistance or blood sugar imbalances. The original recipe does not include ghee, but I find it adds that perfect touch of healthy fats, which is essential for helping to transport nutrients to your cells.

SERVES 4

4 medium zucchini, chopped

3 cups (330 g) string beans, tough ends removed

2 celery ribs, chopped

1 quart (960 ml) water

1 bunch parsley, stems removed

Pinch of sea salt

2 tsp (9 g) ghee (optional)

Place the zucchini, string beans, celery and water in a stockpot. Bring it to a boil, then lower the heat and simmer for about 20 minutes, until the vegetables are softened but not overcooked. Spoon the mixture into a blender. Add the parsley and a pinch of sea salt. Blend until it's liquefied.

The vegetables from one pot will make about two blender batches, depending on how big your blender is. I like to store my broth in a glass mason jar in the refrigerator. To thicken the broth and enhance the healing properties, add a teaspoon of ghee to each blender batch, if desired.

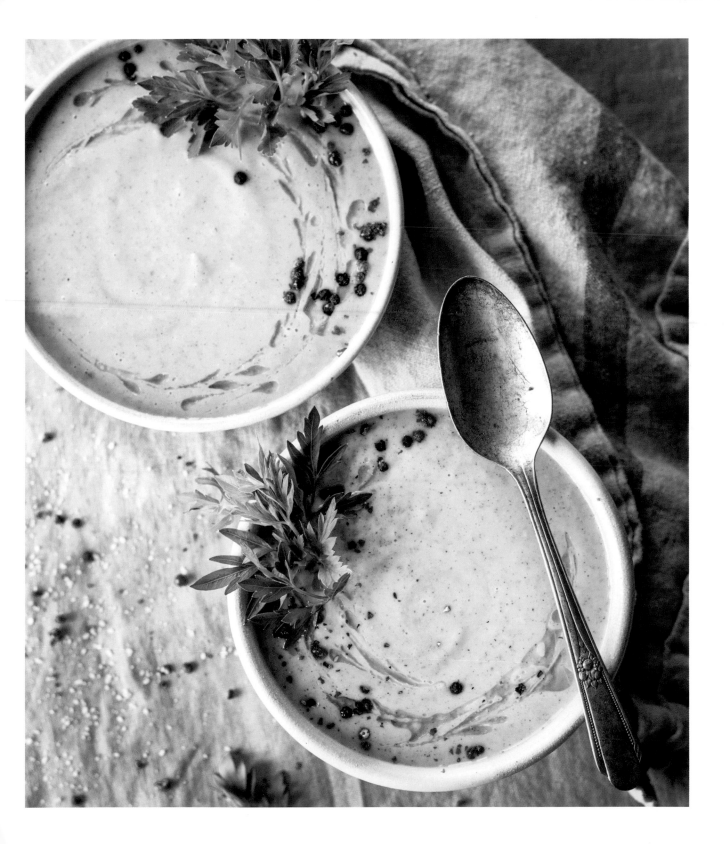

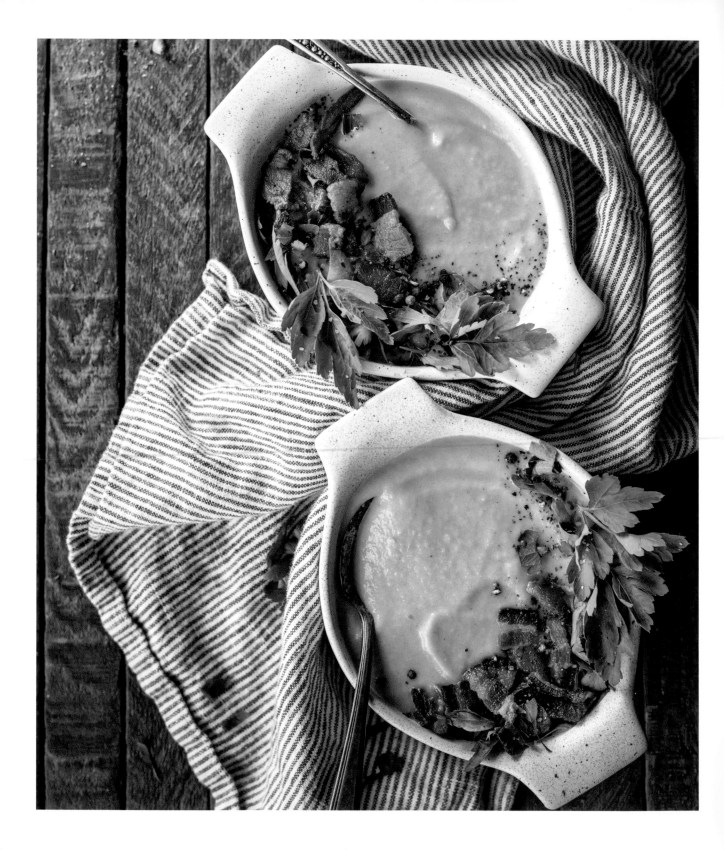

CREAMY CAULIFLOWER SOUP

Cauliflower is making quite the appearance throughout these recipes. As you can see, it's incredibly versatile. Blended and pureed, roasted, and even used as a rice replacement, it's wonderful! You can always forgo the bacon and butter in this recipe and replace it with coconut oil to make it AIP-compliant (Autoimmune Paleo Protocol).

SERVES 4

4 slices bacon, diced

1 tbsp (14 g) grass-fed butter

3 cloves garlic, minced

1 onion, diced

2 carrots, peeled and diced

2 ribs celery, diced

1 large head of cauliflower, stems removed and roughly chopped into florets

1 bay leaf

4 cups (960 ml) chicken or vegetable broth

1 cup (240 ml) full-fat coconut milk

1 tsp sea salt

2 tbsp (8 g) roughly chopped fresh parsley leaves, for garnish

Heat a large stockpot or Dutch oven over medium heat. Add the bacon and cook until it's brown and crispy, about 6 to 8 minutes. Transfer the bacon to a paper towel–lined plate and set it aside. Do not discard the bacon fat.

In the same pot, add the butter, garlic, onion, carrots and celery. Cook, stirring occasionally, until they're slightly soft, about 3 to 4 minutes. Add the cauliflower and bay leaf. Gently stir to combine all the ingredients.

Add the broth and coconut milk, and gently stir to combine them. Cover the pot with a lid and bring it to a boil. Then reduce the heat to a simmer and cook until the cauliflower is fork-tender, about 12 to 15 minutes.

Remove the bay leaf. Season it with sea salt. Transfer the soup to a blender to puree it, or use a hand blender and blend everything together in the pot. Serve garnished with the reserved bacon bits and parsley.

NOTES: If the soup is too thick, you can always add a little more broth or coconut milk until you reach your desired texture.

There should be enough liquid to just cover all the veggies in the pot. More or less broth may be needed, but 5 cups (1.2 L) of liquid was perfect for me. If you need more liquid and don't have any more broth, just use water.

THE BEST COBB SALAD

I could eat this salad for days. It's got the perfect combo of P+F+F (protein, fat and fiber), and it will keep you full for hours. Truth is, this salad can be enjoyed at any meal. I've often enjoyed it for breakfast. I mean, it does have eggs and bacon in it! This is also a great recipe to help you use up different veggies you have on hand. Sliced carrots, celery or cucumber can all work here. Get creative!

SERVES 4

FOR THE DRESSING

¼ cup (60 ml) olive oil

1 tbsp (15 ml) apple cider vinegar

1 tbsp (15 ml) Dijon mustard

1½ tsp (8 ml) honey

¼ tsp sea salt

FOR THE SALAD

4 eggs

Sea salt

6 slices bacon

5 cups (375 g) finely chopped romaine or iceberg lettuce

2 cups (280 g) chopped cooked chicken breasts

1 avocado, peeled, pitted and diced

1 cup (149 g) cherry tomatoes, halved

½ cup (90 g) black olives, pitted

To make the dressing, place the olive oil, vinegar, Dijon mustard, honey and sea salt into a small bowl. Whisk them together until well combined. Alternatively, place the ingredients into a small mason jar and shake well. Set it aside.

To make the salad, place the eggs in a saucepan and fill it with cold water, covering the eggs by an inch (2.5 cm). Add sea salt to the water and bring it to a rolling boil over high heat. Cover the pan with a lid, and remove the eggs from the heat. Let them sit for roughly 10 to 12 minutes. Drain the eggs and when they are completely cooled, peel off the shells and dice the eggs into small pieces. Set them aside.

Place a cast-iron skillet over medium heat. When hot, add the bacon to the skillet. Cook for 15 minutes over medium heat, flipping the slices once halfway through. When cooked, place the bacon on a paper towel to drain and cool. Chop the bacon into small pieces and set them aside.

To assemble the salad, toss together the lettuce and salad dressing in a large bowl. Transfer the lettuce to a platter or leave it in the bowl. Top the lettuce with the chicken, avocado, bacon, eggs, tomatoes and olives.

NOTE: I've often served this salad with the Lemon Tahini Dressing (page 185), and they pair together really well.

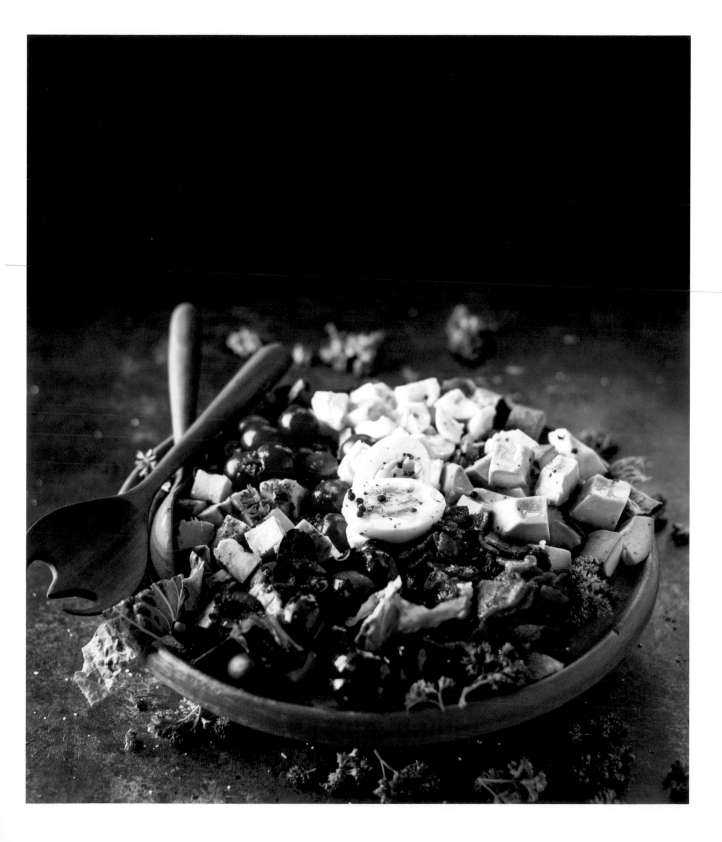

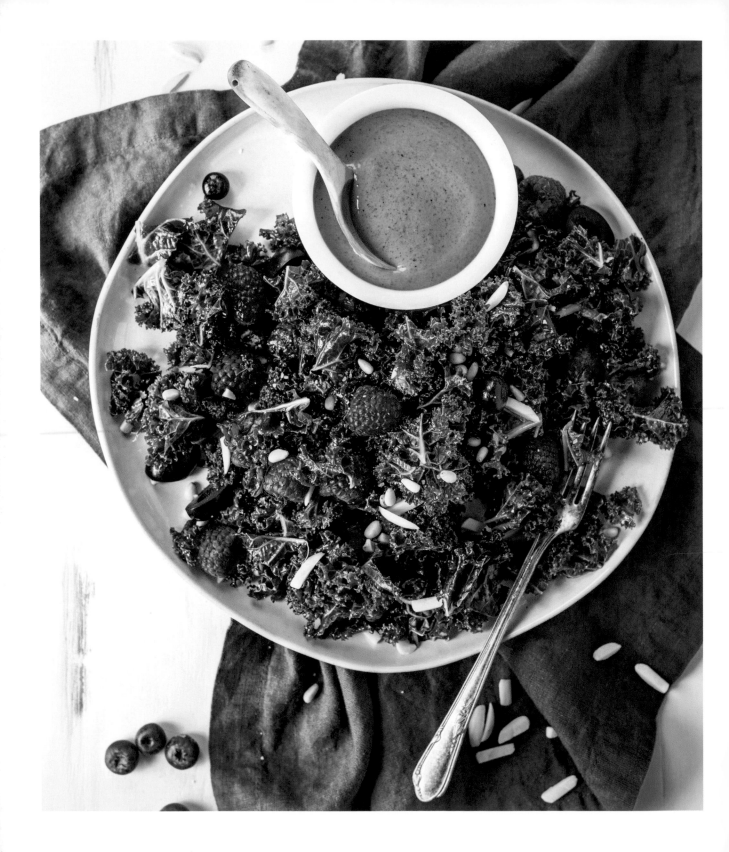

BERRY KALE SALAD

This salad is incredibly refreshing, and it combines the perfect blend of sweet and salty. Kale is often quite bitter, which is why some people tend to avoid eating it. Pairing it with sweet and salty helps to offset the bitterness. Plus, it's loaded with magnesium and is an all-around hormone-loving green—so eat up!

SERVES 4

5–6 cups (335–402 g) kale, chopped

1½ tbsp (23 ml) plus 1 tsp olive oil, divided

¼ tsp sea salt

¾ cup (111 g) fresh blueberries

1 cup (138 g) fresh cherries or raspberries (cherries must be pitted and halved)

¼ cup (34 g) pine nuts

1 tsp slivered almonds

¼ cup (45 g) black olives, roughly chopped (optional)

1 recipe Cherry Berry Vinaigrette (page 186)

Massage the kale by placing it in a bowl, with 1½ tablespoons (23 ml) of olive oil and sea salt. Using your hands, massage the oil and salt into the kale for a good 5 minutes until you reach your desired texture. If you prefer the kale softer, massage it a few minutes longer.

Top the salad with the blueberries, cherries, pine nuts, almonds, olives (if using) and 1 teaspoon of olive oil. Drizzle on the vinaigrette and serve.

AVOCADO, TOMATO & CUCUMBER SALAD

It doesn't get easier than only four ingredients. I often prefer this salad over a green leafy one. The avocado is so creamy, and the tomatoes and cucumbers give an amazing freshness and crunch. The onion adds the perfect bite. When combined with The Simplest Dressing (page 182), you've got a quick and hormone-balancing salad to serve alongside your main meal. If you can tolerate dairy, feel free to crumble on some goat or

sheep feta.

SERVES 2

2 avocados, peeled, pitted and chopped

2 cups (298 g) cherry tomatoes, cut in half

2 cups (266 g) chopped cucumber

1–2 tbsp (10–20 g) finely chopped red onion

1 recipe The Simplest Dressing (page 182)

In a large bowl, add the avocados, tomatoes, cucumber and red onion. Gently mix them together. Drizzle with 2 to 3 tablespoons (30 to 45 ml), or your desired amount, of the dressing. Mix well to combine them. Serve with your main meal and enjoy.

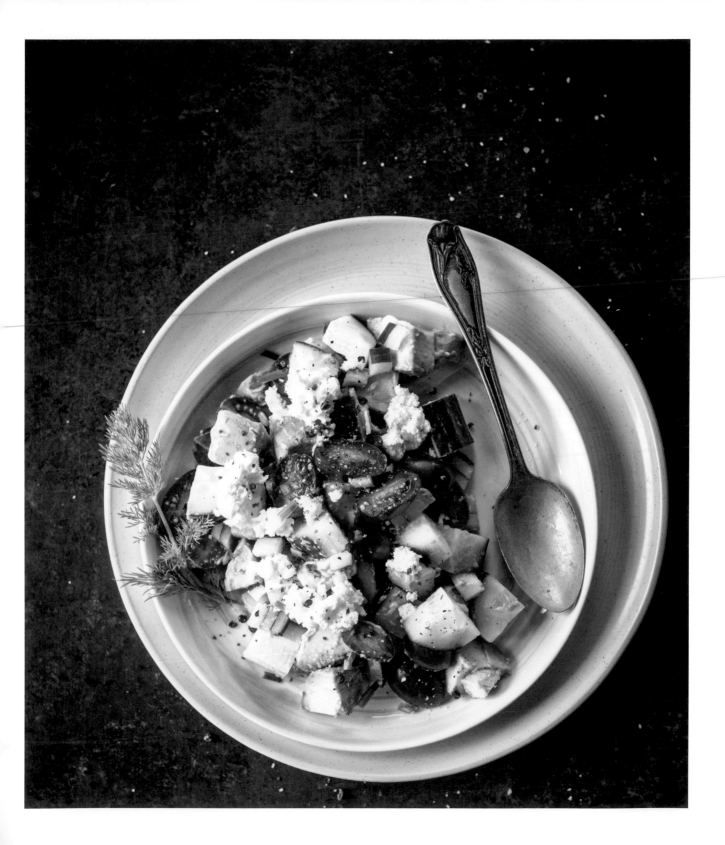

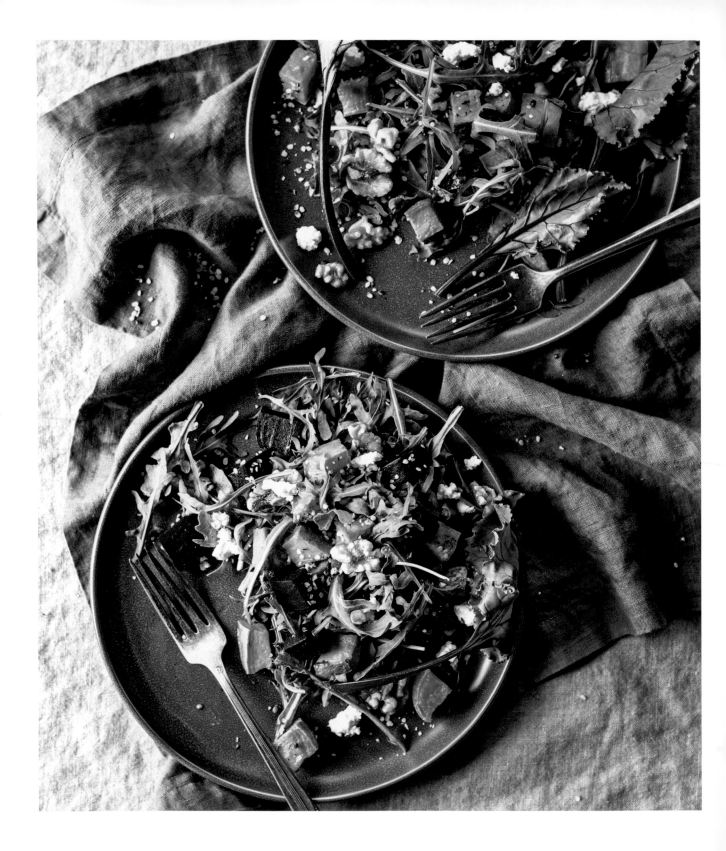

SWEET POTATO, BEET & ARUGULA DETOX SALAD

The combination of sweet potatoes and beets is perfection. If you've been hesitant to go grain-free because you'll miss your carbs, I can promise you this recipe will hit the carb sweet spot! Root vegetables contain more nutrition and minerals than grains, plus they are fiber-rich, which is great for your bowels. This recipe does require some prep. I like to roast extra sweet potatoes and beets earlier in the week so that I can have them on hand to make this salad come the weekend.

SERVES 4 TO 6

2 medium beets

2 medium sweet potatoes

Sea salt

4 cups (120 g) arugula or spinach

¼ cup (29 g) roughly chopped walnuts

1 tbsp (7 g) hemp seeds

¼ cup (38 g) soft goat cheese, crumbled

1 recipe The Simplest Dressing (page 182)

Preheat the oven to 375°F (190°C, or gas mark 5), and cover a baking sheet with parchment paper.

Remove the stems and leaves from the beets, and wash them thoroughly. Wrap them in foil and bake in the oven for about 1 hour, or until the beets are fork-tender. Remove the beets from the foil and let them stand for 15 to 20 minutes, or until they are cool enough to handle. Loosen the skins from the beets and cut them into cubes.

Meanwhile, wash the sweet potatoes, leaving the peel on. Cut them into 1-inch (2.5-cm) pieces, and place the sweet potatoes onto the prepared baking sheet. Sprinkle them with sea salt. Bake for 30 to 40 minutes, or until the sweet potatoes are soft and cooked through.

When your beets and sweet potatoes are roasted and ready to eat, prepare the salad. Add the arugula to a large bowl. Top with the roasted sweet potatoes, beets, walnuts, hemp seeds, and goat cheese, drizzle with the dressing and toss them together to combine.

NOTES: You can simply add a 4- to 6-ounce (113- to 170-g) piece of grilled chicken or salmon to this salad and turn it into a main meal.

Place the foil-wrapped beets on the same tray as the sweet potatoes and roast them at the same time. Be sure to check them at the halfway mark. Sweet potatoes will cook faster, so remove them earlier.

SALAD DRESSINGS AND SIDES

THE SIMPLEST DRESSING

This dressing is fail-proof. It's one of those dressings that works on roasted veggies, on salads and even as a quick-and-simple marinade for chicken or fish.

MAKES 1 SERVING

3 tbsp (45 ml) extra virgin olive oil

1 tbsp (15 ml) balsamic vinegar

Juice of ½ lemon

1 tsp dried oregano

Pinch of sea salt

Add the olive oil, vinegar, lemon juice, oregano and sea salt to a mason jar. Place the lid on the jar and give it a good shake.

NOTE: You can double or triple this recipe and store it in the fridge for later use throughout the week.

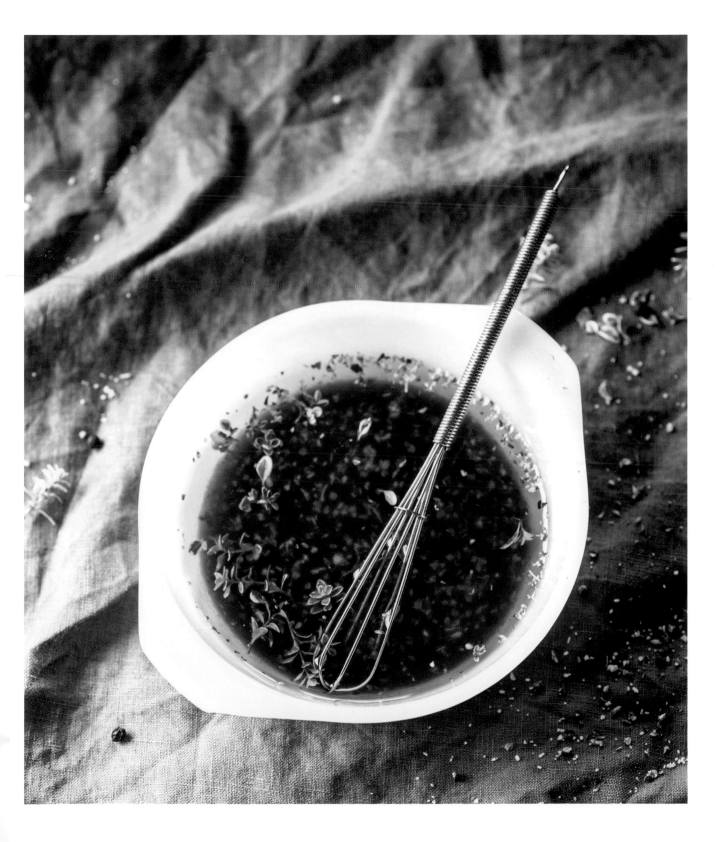

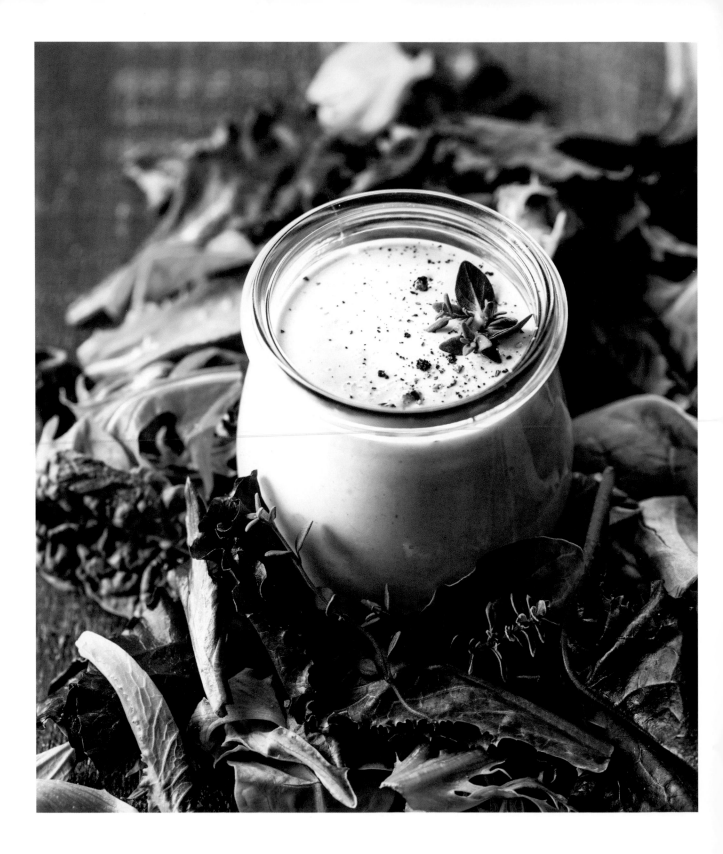

LEMON TAHINI DRESSING

I absolutely love this dressing so much! It works wonderfully as a veggie dip, a sandwich spread, drizzled on roasted veggies and, of course, for salads. Tahini is made from ground sesame seeds, and it is incredibly rich in plant-based calcium.

MAKES 2 TO 2½ CUPS (ABOUT 480 TO 600 ML)

1 cup (240 ml) water, divided

Juice from 1 lemon

1 cup (240 g) raw tahini

2 cloves garlic, roughly chopped

Pinch of cayenne pepper, to taste

1 tsp maple syrup (optional)

1 tbsp (1–3 g) mixed herbs (basil, parsley, oregano, etc.), or to taste

1 tsp dried dulse

½ tsp sea salt

Place ½ cup (120 ml) of water and the lemon juice in a blender or food processor. With the blender or food processor running, gradually add the tahini. Blend, adding additional water to create the desired consistency.

Add the garlic, cayenne pepper, maple syrup (if using), herbs, dulse and sea salt. Blend until it's smooth. Add more water if necessary, for taste or consistency. This dressing will keep in the refrigerator for several days.

CHERRY BERRY VINAIGRETTE

This dressing sings summer. It's so light and refreshing, and it provides you with a healthy dose of antioxidants such as vitamin C.

MAKES 1 SERVING

¼ cup (37 g) fresh blueberries

¼ cup (39 g) fresh pitted cherries or raspberries

1 tbsp (15 ml) fresh lemon juice

Pinch of sea salt

¼ cup (60 ml) olive oil

Add the blueberries, cherries, lemon juice, sea salt and olive oil to a blender or food processor. Combine until it's smooth.

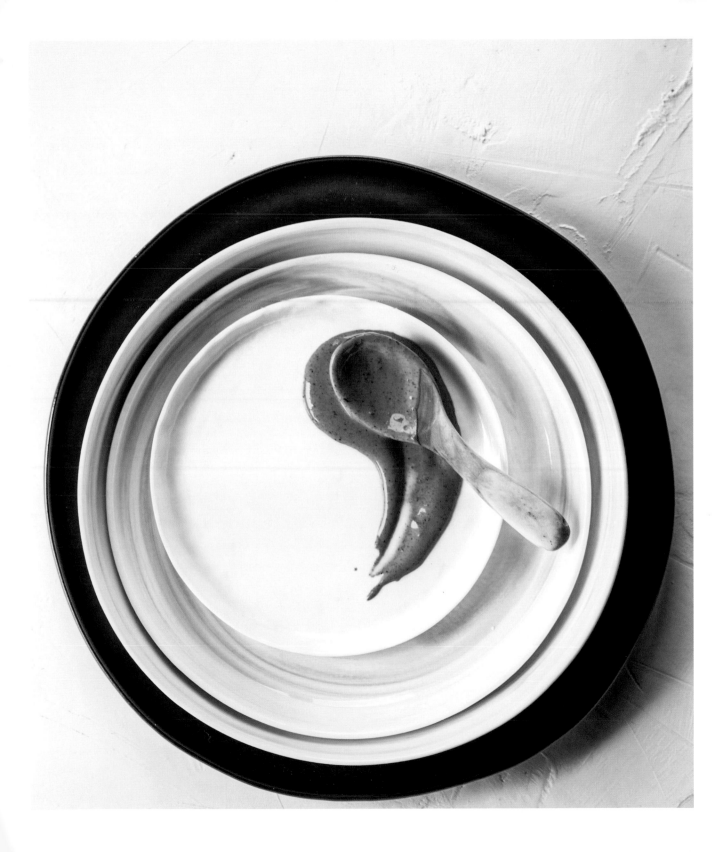

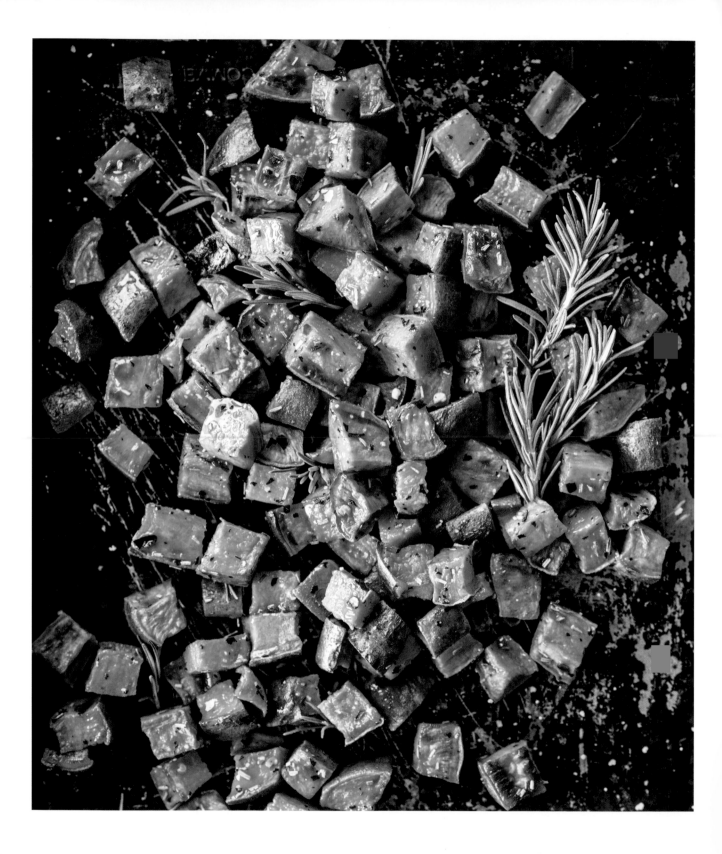

HERBED ROASTED SWEET POTATOES

Sweet potatoes are a regular in our house. You can mash them or roast them. Enjoy them in a sweet or savory dish, or combine them with a variety of herbs for a simple weeknight side dish. I love to make extra of this dish and serve it with scrambled eggs the next morning. Sweet potatoes are rich in fiber, vitamin B_6 and iron. And when you're eliminating grains, they are the perfect starchy veggie to enjoy and indulge in. Oh, and ladies! That B_6 is wonderful for combating period cramps. Feel free to serve these sweet potatoes with a few drizzles of the Lemon Tahini Dressing (page 185).

SERVES 4

2 medium sweet potatoes, chopped into 2-inch (5-cm) cubes

1 tsp dried oregano

1 tsp dried rosemary

1 tsp red pepper flakes

½ tsp sea salt

Preheat the oven to 375°F (190°C, or gas mark 5), and line a large baking sheet with parchment paper.

Place the sweet potato cubes onto the baking sheet. Sprinkle the oregano, rosemary, red pepper flakes and sea salt onto the sweet potato cubes. Using your hands, gently mix the ingredients together. Roast for about 40 to 45 minutes, or until you've reached your desired tenderness and crispness.

ROASTED ASPARAGUS

Asparagus is rich in glutathione, a potent antioxidant that helps the liver detoxify more effectively. Plus, it's an amazing diuretic and supports the kidneys. If you've been feeling a little bloated or holding on to excess water, load up on asparagus to help your body flush out the excess water.

SERVES 4

1 lb (454 g) asparagus spears
1 tbsp (15 ml) olive oil
1 tsp balsamic vinegar
½ tsp sea salt

Preheat the oven to 350°F (175°C, or gas mark 4), and line a baking dish with parchment paper.

Rinse and clean the asparagus spears, and cut off the dry rough ends. Lay the spears across the baking sheet and drizzle them with olive oil, vinegar and sea salt. Roast for about 15 minutes, or until your desired tenderness is reached.

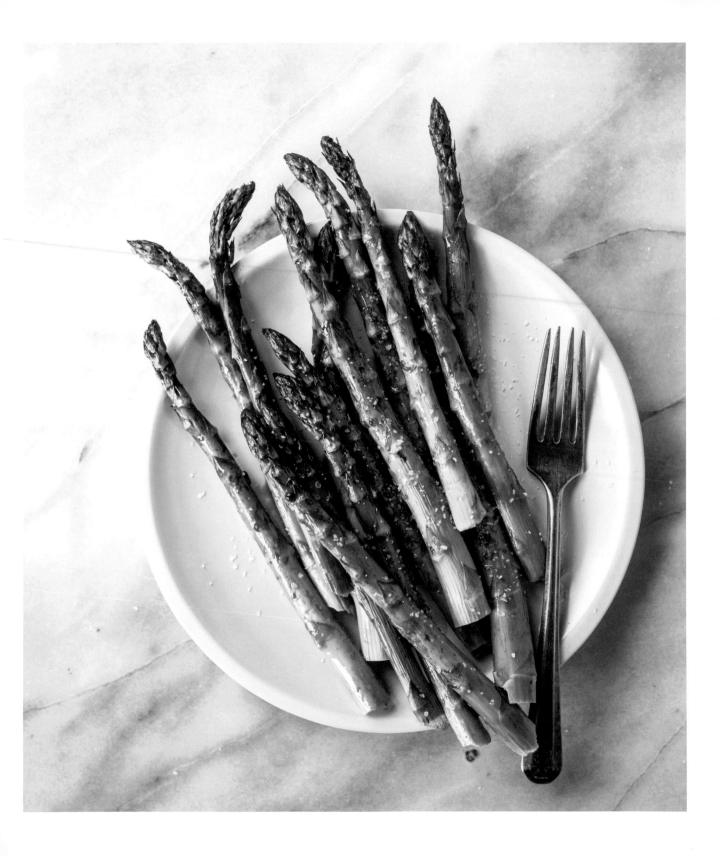

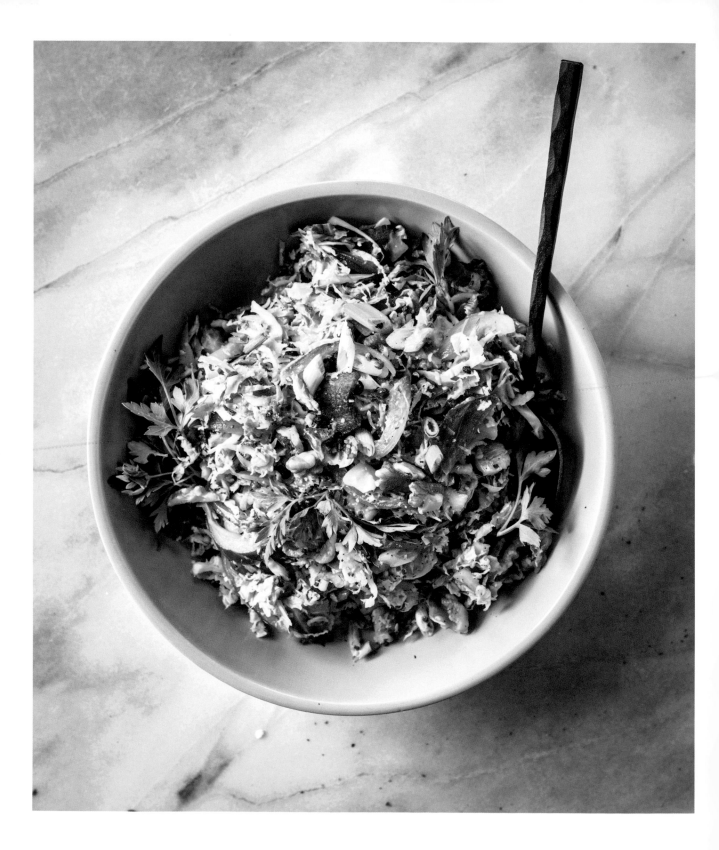

SHAVED BRUSSELS SPROUTS WITH BACON & WALNUTS

I find that Brussels sprouts rank low on the fan-favorite veggie list. I personally love them! From a health perspective, they are one of the top detox-friendly, hormone-optimizing foods. Ever notice that smell when cutting your Brussels sprouts? That's sulfur, and it's amazing for liver detoxification. Plus, these green little gems are loaded with vitamin K, vitamin C, Indole-3-carbinol and sulforaphane—all incredible nutrients for hormonal health, so be sure to eat them on the regular.

SERVES 4

4 slices bacon, cut into ¼-inch (6-mm) pieces

1½ lb (680 g) Brussels sprouts, stems removed

½ cup (80 g) thinly sliced red onion

1½ tsp (5 g) sea salt

2 tbsp (30 ml) sherry vinegar

2 tbsp (8 g) minced Italian parsley

2 tbsp (6 g) minced chives

½ cup (59 g) walnuts or pecans, roughly chopped

Place a skillet over medium heat and toss in the bacon pieces. Cook the bacon, stirring occasionally, until the bits are crispy, 4 to 5 minutes.

While the bacon is crisping in the skillet, shred the Brussels sprouts using the slicing blade of a food processor. If you don't have a food processor, simply slice them thinly with a sharp knife.

Check on the bacon. When it's crispy and cooked through, remove it from the pan using a slotted spoon and transfer it to a plate. Set it aside.

Add the red onion to the skillet and cook it in the bacon grease. Sauté until the onion is soft, about 3 to 4 minutes. Add the shaved Brussels sprouts and season with the sea salt. Stir-fry until the Brussels sprouts are tender, about 5 to 7 minutes.

Turn off the heat, add the sherry vinegar and gently mix it all together. Add the parsley, chives, bacon bits and nuts. Serve alongside your main meal.

GARLICKY CAULIFLOWER RICE

If you've been missing rice, I promise, cauliflower is here to the rescue. This dish is so simple to make, and it can be used in any recipe that calls for rice or fried rice. I like having extras of this recipe on hand throughout the week as it makes the perfect side dish for any meat or fish. Cauliflower is the perfect detox-friendly food. It's rich in vitamin C, which helps with collagen production, and it's loaded with fiber, which is great for gut health.

SERVES 4

1 large head cauliflower

2 tbsp (30 ml) oil (coconut oil, ghee, butter or olive oil work well)

3 cloves garlic, chopped

¼ tsp sea salt

2 tbsp (8 g) roughly chopped fresh parsley

Wash and thoroughly dry the cauliflower, then remove all the greens and cut off the stem. Coarsely chop the cauliflower into florets. Place it in the food processor; you might have to do this in a couple of batches.

Pulse the cauliflower until it resembles rice or couscous—don't overprocess or it will get mushy. Scoop out the cauliflower, set it aside in a bowl and repeat with the remaining cauliflower. If desired, transfer it to a clean towel or paper towel, and squeeze out any excess moisture.

When you have your cauliflower riced, it's easy to cook! Heat a large skillet over medium heat and add the oil to the skillet. When the oil is warm, add the garlic and sauté for 1 minute. Add the cauliflower rice, giving it a quick stir, then cover the skillet with a lid so the cauliflower steams and becomes more tender. Cook for a total of 6 to 8 minutes, then season it with the sea salt and parsley.

You can store uncooked cauliflower rice in the freezer for up to 1 month.

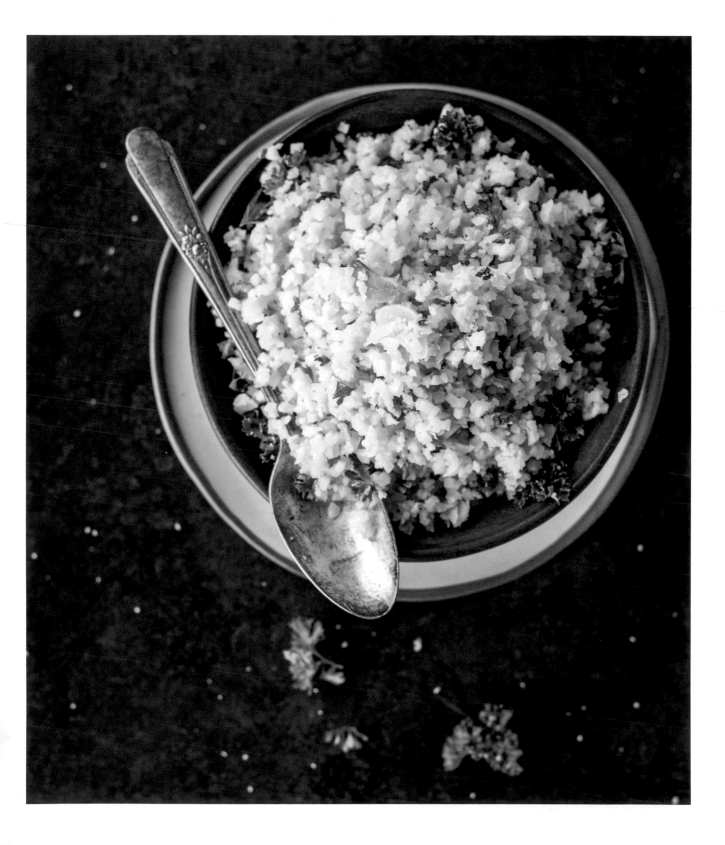

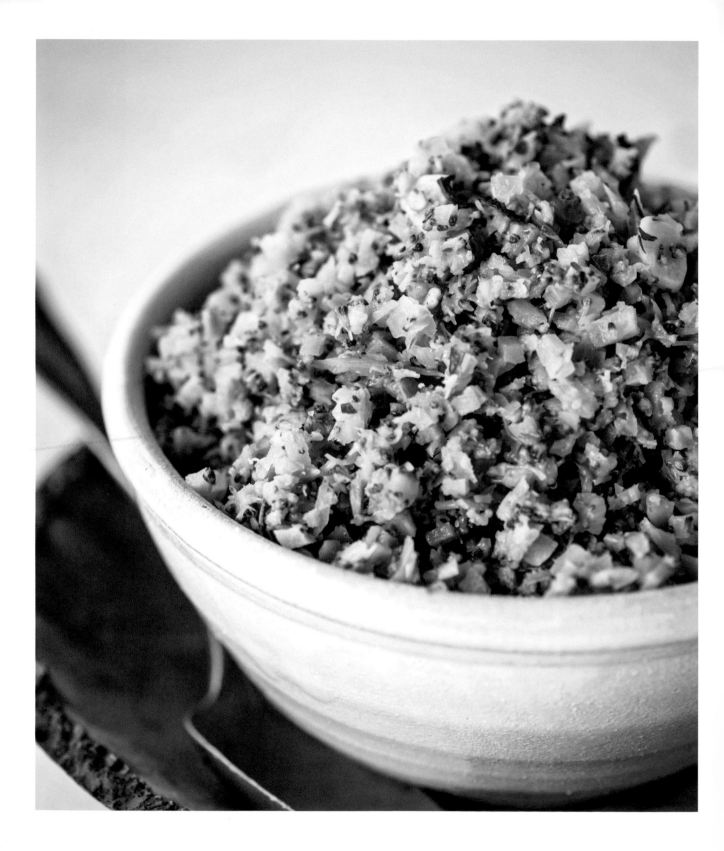

BROCCOLI RICE

We all know that broccoli is a nutritional powerhouse, but I can honestly admit that it's not my favorite vegetable. Let's face it, eating it raw or simply boiling it doesn't do it any favors. Enter broccoli rice—one of my favorite ways to enjoy this green superfood, support liver detoxification and love on my hormones. Feel free to add your favorite herbs and spices to this dish. I often sauté my broccoli rice with some onion powder and a pinch of red pepper flakes for some extra spice.

SERVES 4

2 heads broccoli, roughly chopped

2 tbsp (27 g) coconut oil or grass-fed butter

Sea salt, herbs and spices

Place the broccoli in the bowl of a food processor and pulse until tiny pieces of "rice" form. In a skillet, heat the oil over medium heat. Add the riced broccoli and lightly cook for 5 to 7 minutes, until it's softened. Season with sea salt and your favorite herbs and spices.

CREAMY CAULIFLOWER "NO POTATO" SALAD

But seriously . . . what would life be like without cauliflower! This recipe is so damn good I've eaten the entire bowl many times during recipe testing. I think the reason I love it most is the fresh dill—which is one of my absolute favorite herbs. And talk about P+F+F (protein, fat and fiber) perfection. The eggs, the cauliflower and the delicious fats from the tahini make this recipe a hormone-loving dream! Serve alongside a slice of Grain-Free Almond Flour Bread (page 100) for a delicious lunch or dinner.

SERVES 6

TAHINI DILL DRESSING

¼ cup (60 g) tahini

1 tbsp (15 ml) olive oil

1 tbsp (15 ml) apple cider vinegar

2 tbsp (30 ml) fresh lemon juice

1 tbsp (15 ml) Dijon mustard

2 tbsp (8 g) chopped fresh dill

2 tbsp (6 g) chopped fresh chives

1 shallot, roughly chopped

2 cloves garlic

1 tsp sea salt

⅓ cup (80 ml) water

⅓ cup (53 g) roughly chopped pickles (I used gherkins.)

SALAD

5 cups (500 g) cauliflower florets

3 eggs

½ cup (51 g) chopped celery

¼ cup (12 g) chopped green onion

¼ cup (40 g) chopped red onion

2 tbsp (8 g) chopped fresh dill

To make the dressing, in a food processor, combine the tahini, olive oil, vinegar, lemon juice, mustard, dill, chives, shallot, garlic, salt and water. Process until it's smooth. Add the pickles and pulse a few times to combine them. Transfer the dressing to a bowl and refrigerate.

To make the salad, bring a large pot of water to a boil. Add the cauliflower florets and cook until they're tender, but still firm, about 15 minutes. Drain the cauliflower and run it under cold water to cool off. Drain it thoroughly, then place it in a large bowl. If you prefer smaller pieces of cauliflower, chop them smaller now before adding them to the bowl. I tend to chop mine fairly small.

Place the eggs in a saucepan and cover them with cold water. Bring the water to a boil, let the eggs boil over the burner for 2 minutes, then cover the pan with a lid and remove the eggs from the heat. Let the eggs rest in the hot water for 12 to 14 minutes to cook through. Remove them from the hot water, cool, peel, chop, then transfer the eggs to the bowl with the cauliflower.

Add the celery, green onion, red onion and dill. Mix to combine them. Add the dressing and mix thoroughly. You can enjoy this salad right away, or place it in the fridge and let it chill, then serve.

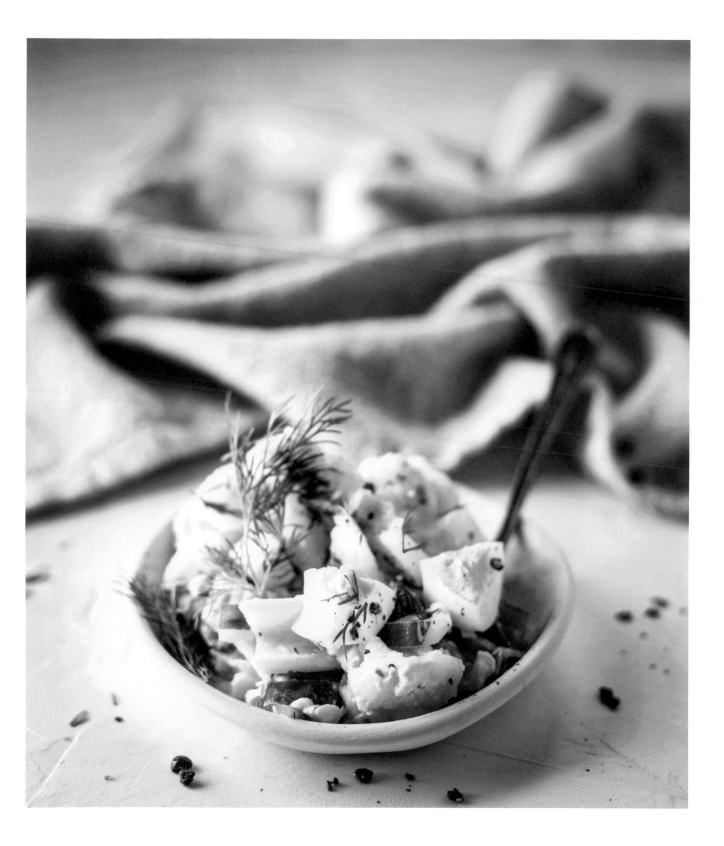

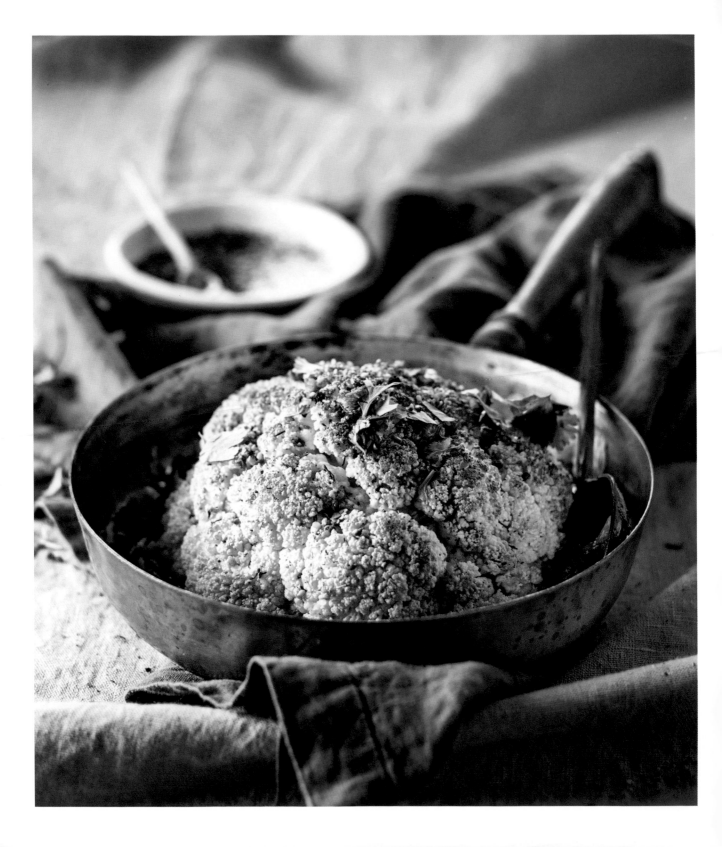

WHOLE ROASTED CAULIFLOWER WITH ZA'ATAR GHEE

There are so many ways to enjoy cauliflower, but this way is my absolute favorite. The texture of the cauliflower is just so good and buttery, and you can get creative using all kinds of marinades or sauces, such as pesto, leftover tomato sauce or even the lemon Dijon chicken marinade (page 120). Alternatively, you can serve your sauces or marinades as a dip. Cauliflower is a hormone-balancing superfood. It contains lots of fiber and phytonutrients that support the detoxification of harmful estrogens. I have a feeling this will become your new favorite way to enjoy cauliflower!

SERVES 4

1 whole head of cauliflower

¼ cup (60 ml) extra virgin olive oil, avocado oil or melted ghee

2 tsp (6 g) sea salt

2 tbsp (22 g) Lee's Ghee Za'atar Star (optional)

Preheat the oven to 375°F (190°C, or gas mark 5), and place a rack in the middle position.

To prepare the cauliflower, you want to remove the core/stem but keep the entire cauliflower intact. Trim away the leaves at the bottom of the cauliflower head as well as the tough core, being careful to keep the head intact. Rinse and dry the cauliflower, and place it in a bowl or on a cutting board. Drizzle the olive oil all over the cauliflower, top and bottom. Sprinkle with the sea salt. Rub the oil and salt all over the head until it's well coated.

Place the cauliflower, florets side up, on a cast-iron skillet, and cover it tightly with aluminum foil. Put the skillet on the middle rack in the oven and cook for 30 minutes, covered. Alternatively, if you do not have a cast-iron pan, place the cauliflower on a baking sheet lined with parchment paper and cover the entire tray with foil. After 30 minutes, remove the foil from the skillet or tray. Roast for 1 hour in the oven.

Ten minutes before the cooking time is up, remove the cauliflower from the oven and spread on the za'atar ghee. Place it back in the oven for the remaining 10 minutes. Alternatively, you can omit this step and eat as is or served with a touch of sea salt and cracked black pepper.

After 1 hour, the cauliflower should be golden-brown on the outside and tender on the inside. A knife should slide in and out quite easily. Transfer the cauliflower head to a platter, carve and serve.

CAULIFLOWER GNOCCHI WITH HOME-MADE ROASTED CHERRY TOMATO SAUCE

Let me just count the many ways to use cauliflower. Honestly, I lost count! There's just too many. I live in Canada and we don't have a Trader Joe's, and we can't get our hands on the extremely popular Trader Joe's Cauliflower Gnocchi. So, after many failed attempts trying to head to the United States to get this gnocchi, which was always sold out, I decided to make my own. All I gotta say is, Trader Joe's has got nothing on me. I suggest you triple this recipe—because it's that good—and freeze extras for future use.

SERVES 4

FOR THE SAUCE

4 cups (596 g) cherry tomatoes

6 cloves garlic, left whole with peel off

3 tbsp (45 ml) olive oil

1 tsp dried oregano

1 tsp dried basil

½ tsp sea salt, plus more to taste

FOR THE CAULIFLOWER GNOCCHI

4 cups (400 g) cauliflower

¾ cup (96 g) cassava flour

1 tsp garlic powder

1 tsp onion powder

½ tsp sea salt

1–2 tbsp (15–30 ml) olive oil, for drizzling

To make the sauce, preheat the oven to 375°F (190°C, or gas mark 5), and line a baking sheet with parchment paper. Rinse and wash the cherry tomatoes, then place them on the baking sheet, with the garlic cloves, olive oil, oregano, basil and sea salt. Using your hands, give everything a mix, making sure the tomatoes are coated well with the olive oil.

Place the baking sheet in the oven and bake for 25 minutes, or until the tomatoes start to shrivel. When cooked, place everything into a food processor and blend until they're well combined. Season with extra sea salt if desired. Set it aside.

To make the cauliflower gnocchi, preheat the oven to 425°F (220°C, or gas mark 7). Start first by turning the cauliflower into rice by blending it in your food processor. Place a steamer basket over boiling water and steam the cauliflower rice for about 5 minutes until it's soft. Alternatively, you can boil the rice for 3 to 4 minutes, then rinse and drain it.

Place the cooked cauliflower into a dish towel, cheesecloth or nut milk bag. Wring out all the water. Squeeze it until all the excess water is out and the cauliflower looks dry. You should end up with roughly 1½ cups (about 270 g).

In a food processor, blend together the cauliflower, cassava flour, garlic powder, onion powder and sea salt. You may have to add more cassava flour to get the dough to be kneadable and dense. Ultimately, you don't want a wet dough, but a dry and kneadable dough.

Roll the dough into a large ball, then separate it into four equal parts. Roll out the dough into ¾-inch (2-cm) diameter tubes on a surface dusted lightly with cassava flour. Cut the tubes of dough into 1-inch (2.5-cm) gnocchi pieces.

Bring a large pot of water to a boil and drop the gnocchi in. When the gnocchi have risen to the surface, remove them with a slotted spoon and place them on a baking sheet lined with parchment paper. Drizzle the gnocchi lightly with olive oil.

Place the gnocchi in the oven at 425°F (220°C, or gas mark 7) for 25 minutes, making sure to turn them halfway through. You want the gnocchi to turn golden-brown on each side. If you prefer them crispier, cook longer.

Alternatively, instead of baking in the oven, you can heat a large cast-iron pan over medium heat and add 2 tablespoons (30 ml) of olive oil. Cook the gnocchi in the pan for 5 to 7 minutes until they're golden-brown. You may need to cook them in batches and continue to add olive oil to prevent sticking.

Serve the gnocchi with the roasted cherry tomato sauce and your choice of protein for a complete meal.

NOTE: I've enjoyed gnocchi alongside Meatloaf Muffins (page 127), Lemon Dijon Chicken Thighs (page 120) or my Cast-Iron Roasted Chicken Thighs with Veggies (page 128). In place of the tomato sauce you can also use walnut pesto (page 143). The possibilities are endless. ENJOY!

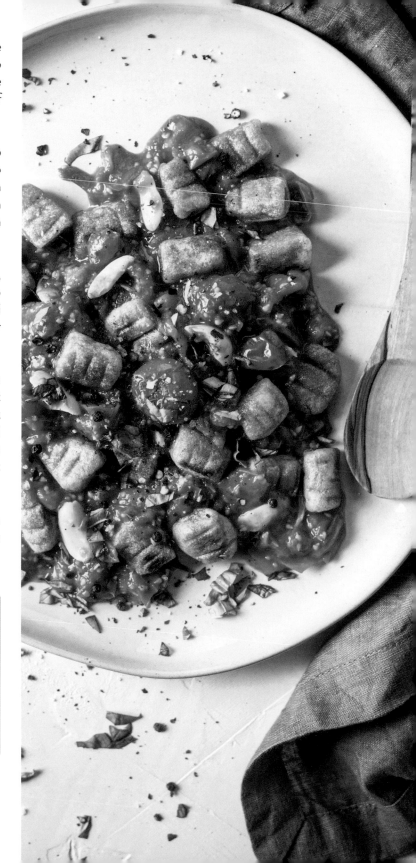

DESSERTS AND TREATS

GUT GUMMIES

Collagen and gelatin have made their way onto the health scene quite a bit in the past two years. You don't need to consume bone broth just to get the benefits—although, bone broth is life! Gelatin is an incredibly healing food, and it is loaded with amino acids that help heal the gut. I love cherries, and I figured why not make cherry gut gummies as a gut-healing, therapeutic treat?! I like using molds for these gut gummies. Alternatively, you can pour the mixture into a brownie pan and when they are set, you can cut them into squares.

MAKES 12 OR MORE

3 tbsp (45 ml) lemon juice

¾ cup (180 ml) water

1 cup (154 g) fresh or frozen cherries (pits removed if using fresh)

¼ cup (60 ml) maple syrup

1 tsp ground ginger

¼ cup (35 g) gelatin

In a blender, add the lemon juice, water and cherries. Blend on high until they're well combined.

Pour this mixture into a saucepan. Turn the heat to medium-low, and whisk in the maple syrup, ginger and gelatin. Continue whisking the mixture for a good 5 minutes, until no clumps remain and you have a thin mixture.

If you are using molds, place your molds onto a baking sheet for easy transfer to the fridge. Trust me on this one! It can get messy! Carefully pour the mixture into a mold or brownie dish, and set it in the fridge to firm up for 1 hour.

NOTE: If using a mold, I suggest putting the gummies in the freezer for 5 minutes before serving. This extra step helps pop the gummies out of the mold easily.

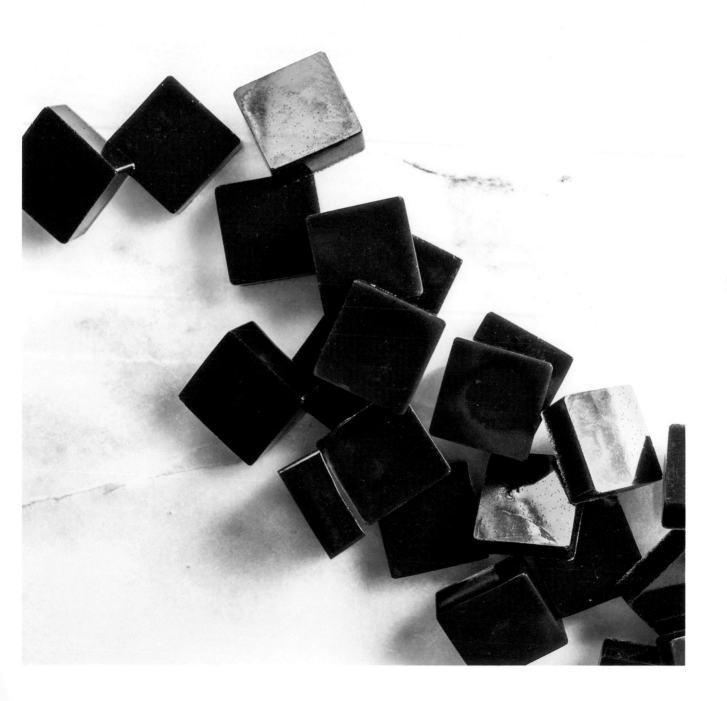

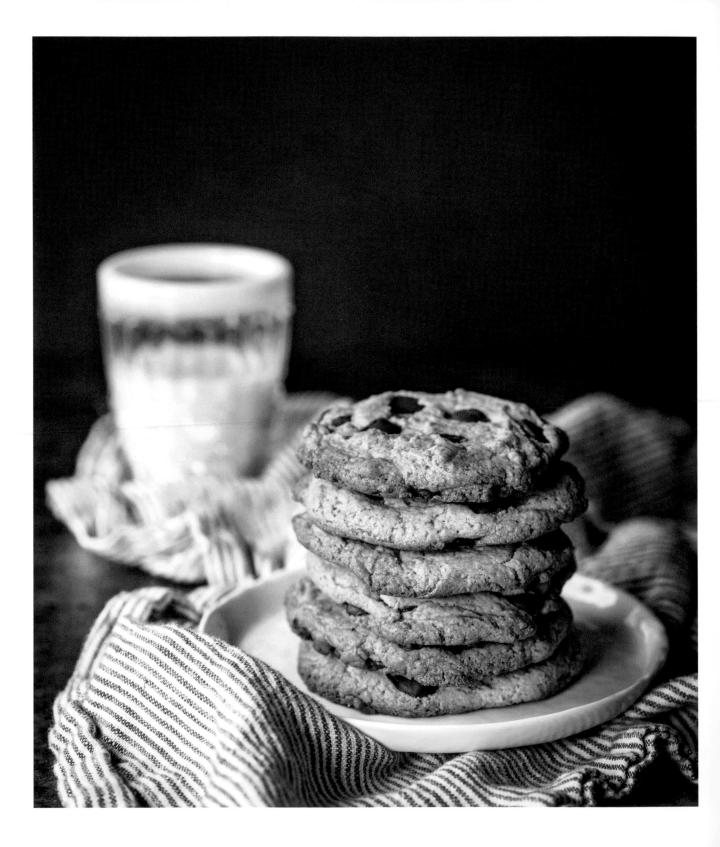

COLLAGEN TAHINI CHOCOLATE CHIP COOKIES (AKA BEST-EVER COOKIES)

If you're looking for a staple chocolate chip cookie, this is it! These cookies are chewy, soft and perfectly sweet. I love using monk fruit as a sweetener as it doesn't spike blood sugar and it's zero calories—bonus! Coconut sugar would work well here, too. Tahini is loaded with calcium, which is great for supporting bone density, and it lends these cookies the perfect texture and softness. I bet you can't eat just one!

MAKES 12 TO 15 COOKIES

1 cup (95 g) almond flour

1½ tbsp (9 g) collagen powder

1 tsp baking soda

¼ cup (48 g) monk fruit or coconut sugar

½ tsp sea salt

1 cup (240 g) tahini

¼ cup (60 ml) maple syrup

1 tsp vanilla extract

1 egg

¾ cup (235 g) dairy-free chocolate chips

Preheat the oven to 350°F (175°C, or gas mark 4), and line a baking sheet with parchment paper.

Add the almond flour, collagen powder, baking soda, monk fruit and sea salt to a large bowl. Mix well. Then add the tahini, maple syrup, vanilla and egg. Mix the ingredients together well. Add the chocolate chips and gently mix until they're combined.

Using your hands, shape the dough into 12 cookies. I sometimes get 15 cookies out of this batter; it just depends on how large or small you make them. Roll each cookie into a ball in your hands, then gently flatten it into a cookie shape and place it on the baking sheet. Repeat this process for all of the cookies. Be sure to leave enough room on your baking sheet between each cookie; they do expand while baking.

Bake in the oven for 12 to 15 minutes: 12 minutes will give you a softer cookie, and 15 minutes will add a bit more of a crunch. When baked to your preference, remove the baking sheet from the oven and let it cool for 15 minutes before serving.

DOUBLE CHOCOLATE CHIP MUFFINS

Oh, chocolate, how I love thee! Fun fact—chocolate is incredibly rich in magnesium, an important mineral needed for detoxification. It's important to choose quality chocolate when it comes to treating yourself. I prefer cacao powder; cocoa tends to be high in sugar and is often processed. Enjoy these chocolatey-gems guilt-free and keep the sugar content low with a sweetener such as monk fruit, or opt for coconut sugar or maple sugar.

MAKES 9 MUFFINS

2 large eggs, at room temperature

¼ cup (60 ml) melted coconut oil

2 tbsp (32 g) sunflower seed butter

¼ cup (48 g) monk fruit, coconut sugar or maple sugar, or to taste

1 sifted cup (140 g) cacao powder

1 tsp baking soda

1 tsp sea salt, or to taste

¼ cup (60 ml) coconut cream

¼ cup (60 ml) hot water, plus more as needed

1 tsp vanilla extract

½ cup (157 g) dark chocolate chips or chunks, divided

Preheat the oven to 350°F (175°C, or gas mark 4). Line a muffin tin with 9 muffin liners.

In a large bowl, whisk together the eggs, coconut oil and sunflower seed butter with a fork. Add the monk fruit and mix it in thoroughly.

Stir in the cacao powder, baking soda and sea salt until they're well combined. Your batter will become dry, which is okay. Add the coconut cream, followed by the hot water and vanilla, and stir until the mixture is fluid again. If the mixture is still thick, add hot water one spoonful at a time, mixing it in completely until the batter becomes fluid and cake batter–like.

Give it a taste—don't eat it all!—and adjust the salt or sweetness as needed. Mix in half of the chocolate chips. Distribute the batter into the muffin pan, filling the 9 cups. Top each muffin with 2 to 3 pieces of the remaining chocolate chips.

Bake for 18 to 20 minutes, until the muffins have risen slightly and look firm. Remove the muffins from the oven and let them cool completely before handling.

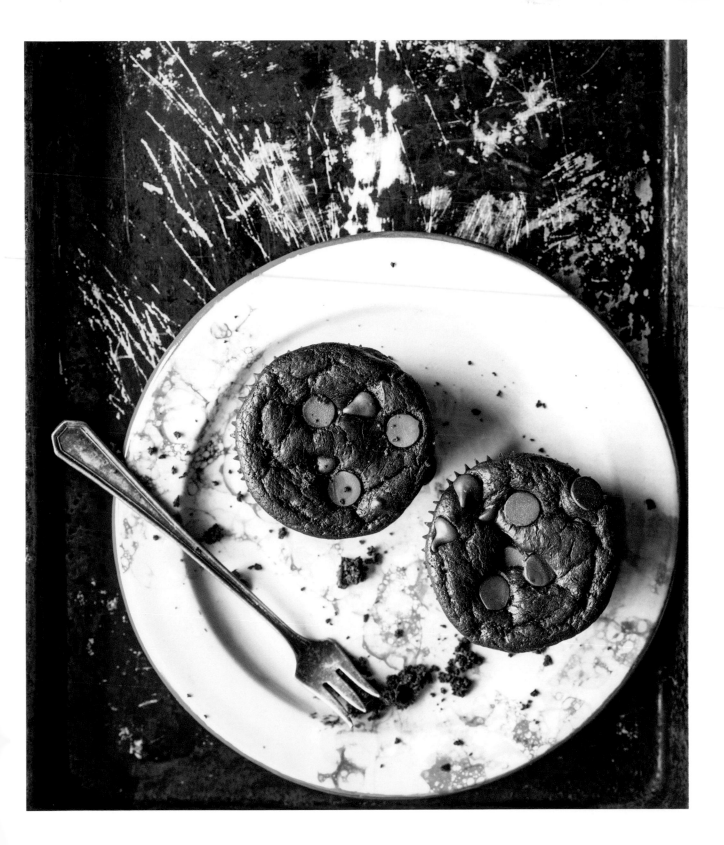

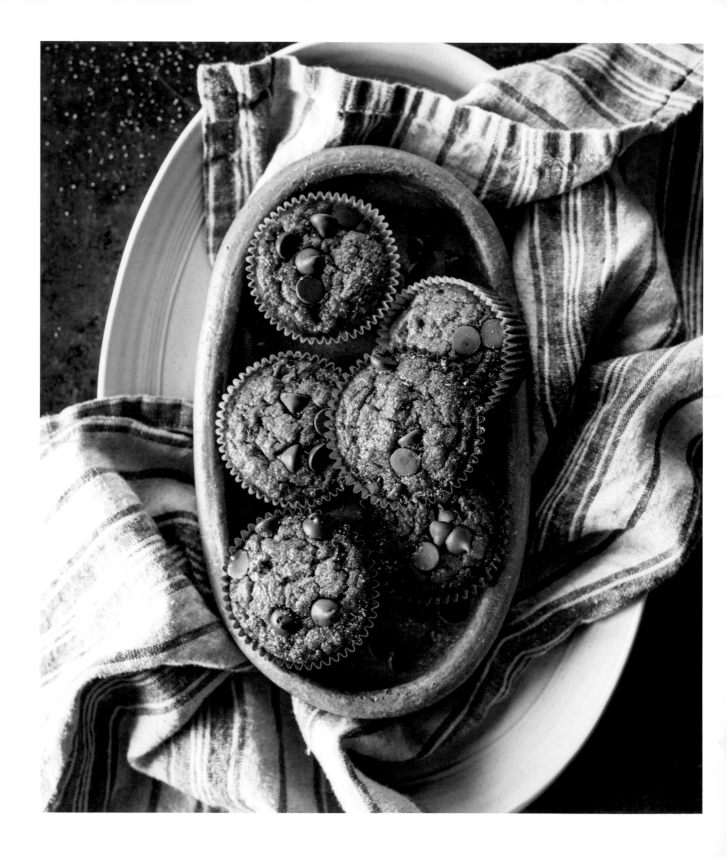

GRAIN-FREE BANANA CHOCOLATE CHIP MUFFINS

Often my Saturday nights are spent baking. These delicious muffins were created on one of those lazy Saturday evenings. Funny to think that ten years ago I was getting dressed up to go out and party at 9 p.m., and nowadays I'm baking grain-free muffins on a Saturday and dreaming up all kinds of grain-free ideas. These fluffy and perfectly sweet muffins just hit the spot, and they are incredibly easy to whip up.

MAKES 12 MUFFINS

2 ripe bananas

4 eggs

1 tsp vanilla extract

¼ cup (60 ml) maple syrup (optional)

½ cup (110 g) coconut oil, melted and cooled is a must

½ cup (60 g) tapioca flour

½ cup (56 g) coconut flour

1 tsp baking soda

1 tsp cinnamon

¼ tsp sea salt

⅓ cup (105 g) chocolate chips, plus more for topping

Preheat the oven to 350°F (175°C, or gas mark 4). Line a 12-cup muffin tin and set it aside.

In a medium-sized bowl, add the bananas and mash them well. Add the eggs and whisk them together with the bananas. Add the vanilla, maple syrup (if using) and the cooled coconut oil, mixing thoroughly.

Add the tapioca flour, coconut flour, baking soda, cinnamon and sea salt to the bowl. Mix until they're well combined. Stir in the chocolate chips. Scoop the batter into the prepared muffins cups. Fill them about three-quarters of the way full. Drop a few extra chocolate chips over top.

Bake for 25 to 28 minutes, or until the muffins are cooked through. Let the muffins cool for about 10 minutes before removing them from the tin.

ALMOND BUTTER FAT BOMBS

So, you go sugar-free or low-carb for a while and then—BAM—one bite of a sweet cake or cookie or piece of bread and your cravings come back full force! Ever notice that? It's normal. Sugar triggers pleasure receptors in your brain, and that causes you to want more and more and more. That's why I like to keep my intake low and opt for sugar-free treats and fat bombs. These delicious, almond butter fat bombs hit the spot without a sugar high, and they leave me feeling satisfied!

MAKES 10 TO 12 FAT BOMBS

¾ cup (156 g) cacao butter, cut into small chunks

2 tbsp (27 g) coconut oil or ghee

3 tbsp (18 g) raw cacao powder

3 heaping tbsp (about 54 g) crunchy or smooth almond butter

¼ tsp vanilla extract

Pinch of sea salt

2 tbsp (24 g) monk fruit, Swerve or liquid stevia, or to taste (optional)

½ cup (42 g) coconut chips, roughly chopped or broken into small pieces (chopped nuts would work well, too)

Line a large muffin tin with silicone liners or parchment baking cups. Over a double boiler, melt the cacao butter and coconut oil together. As they start to melt, add the cacao powder and almond butter, gently stirring everything together.

Add the vanilla, sea salt and sweetener of choice, if using. When melted, remove it from the heat and stir in the coconut chips. Pour the mixture into the silicone muffin molds, filling them just one-quarter of the way.

Place the muffin tin in the freezer for 1 hour to set. Then remove it from the freezer when you're ready to eat. If you are using the silicone molds, the fat bombs pop right out with ease!

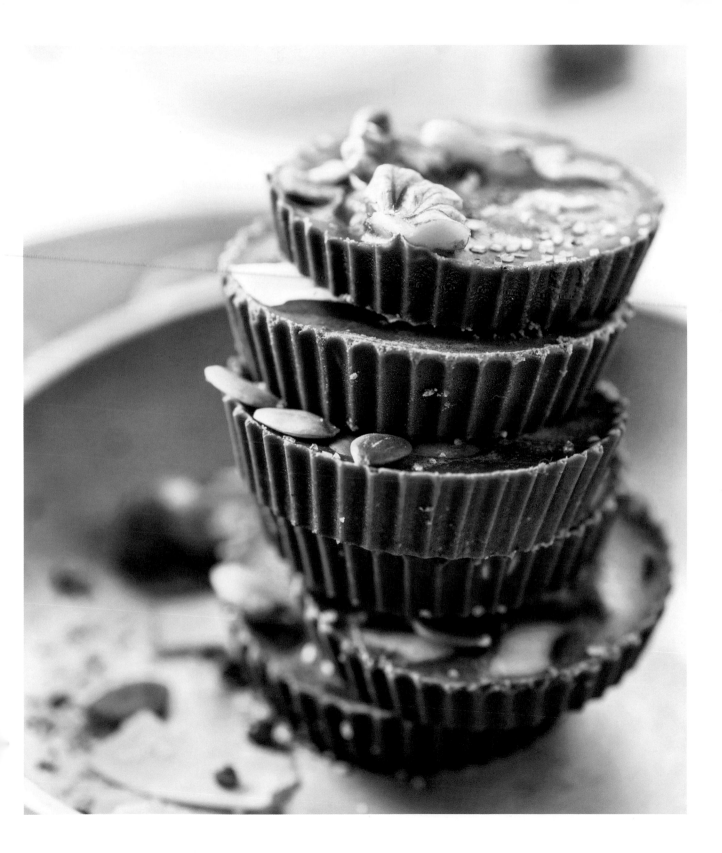

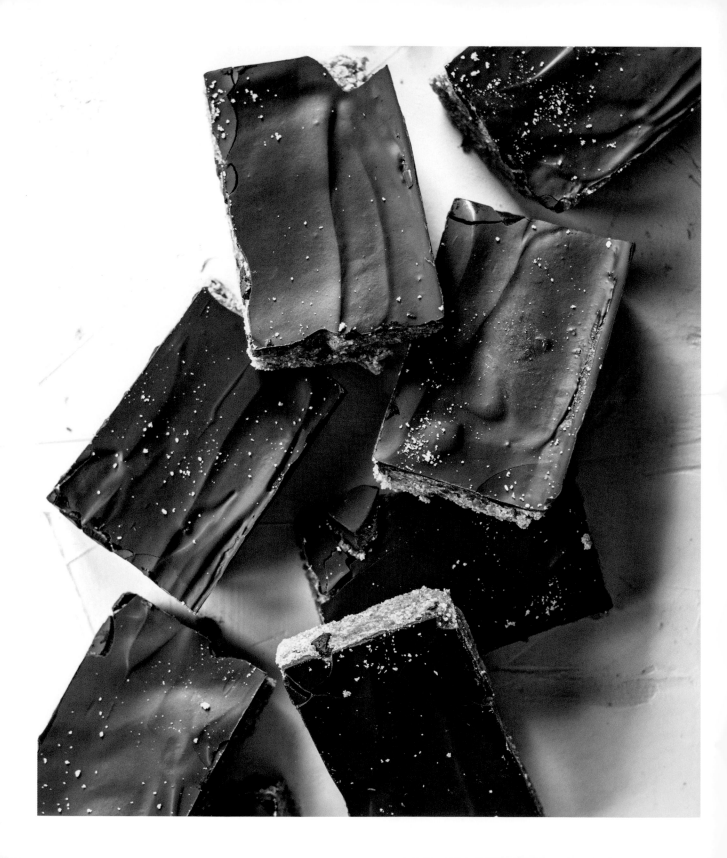

NO-BAKE SUNFLOWER BARS

There is nothing better than a no-bake dessert! These sun butter bars are low in sugar and loaded with healthy fats. Plus, that hit of chocolate on top is perfection. If you're looking to add some protein to this recipe, experiment with ½ cup (56 g) of coconut flour and ½ cup (54 g) of your favorite protein powder. I personally love PurePaleo Protein grass-fed beef from Designs for Health.

MAKES 12 BARS

1 cup (112 g) coconut flour, sifted

1 cup (95 g) almond flour

⅓–½ cup (64–96 g) monk fruit or coconut sugar, or to taste

½ tsp sea salt

½ tsp vanilla extract

½ tsp ground cinnamon

1 cup (258 g) sunflower seed butter or almond butter

¼–½ cup (60–120 ml) almond milk, plus more if needed

½ cup (157 g) dairy-free chocolate chips

1 tsp coconut oil

In a large mixing bowl, combine the coconut flour, almond flour, monk fruit, sea salt, vanilla and cinnamon. Mix together until they're well combined. Add the sunflower seed butter and stir until it's fully incorporated. The batter should be quite crumbly. Add the almond milk, 1 tablespoon (15 ml) at a time, until a very dense batter is formed. You may need roughly ¼ cup (60 ml) of almond milk or more to get the right consistency.

Press the batter firmly into an 8 x 8-inch (20 x 20-cm) baking dish lined with parchment paper and set it aside.

Over a double boiler, melt together the chocolate chips with the coconut oil. When melted, pour it over the bars and smooth over. Refrigerate for at least 1 hour, then cut it into bars.

NO-BAKE PEPPERMINT CHOCOLATE CHEESECAKE

I'm a baking enthusiast and nothing makes me happier than spending time in my kitchen whipping up Paleo treats. If you're looking to wow your guests at a birthday party or event, make them this cake. They. Will. Love. You. Top off this delicious cake with some fresh fruit, chocolate shavings or shredded coconut, and you got yourself a beauty!

SERVES 10

FOR THE CRUST

1½ cups (126 g) large unsweetened coconut chips

½ cup (56 g) coconut flour

½ cup (120 ml) melted coconut oil

3 tbsp (18 g) cacao powder

⅓ cup (80 ml) raw honey or maple syrup

FOR THE FILLING

3 cups (438 g) raw cashews, soaked overnight or for at least 2 hours

1 cup (240 ml) coconut cream, from the can

½ cup (120 ml) melted coconut oil

½ cup (120 ml) raw honey or maple syrup

½ cup (48 g) cacao powder

1 tbsp (15 ml) peppermint extract, or less to taste

Chocolate shavings, coconut chips or fresh berries, for garnish (optional)

To make the crust, in a mixing bowl, combine the coconut chips, coconut flour, coconut oil, cacao powder and raw honey. Mix together until they're well combined. Press the mixture into a 9-inch (23-cm) springform pan to form a crust, then place it in the freezer while you make the filling.

To make the filling, drain and rinse the soaked cashews. Combine the cashews, coconut cream and coconut oil in a food processor. Process until it's smooth and creamy. Add the honey, cacao powder and peppermint extract. Process until it's smooth.

Spread the filling over the crust. Place the cheesecake back in the freezer for about 30 minutes, or until it's set. Top with chocolate shavings, coconut chips or fresh berries, if using. Store leftovers in an airtight container in the refrigerator or freezer.

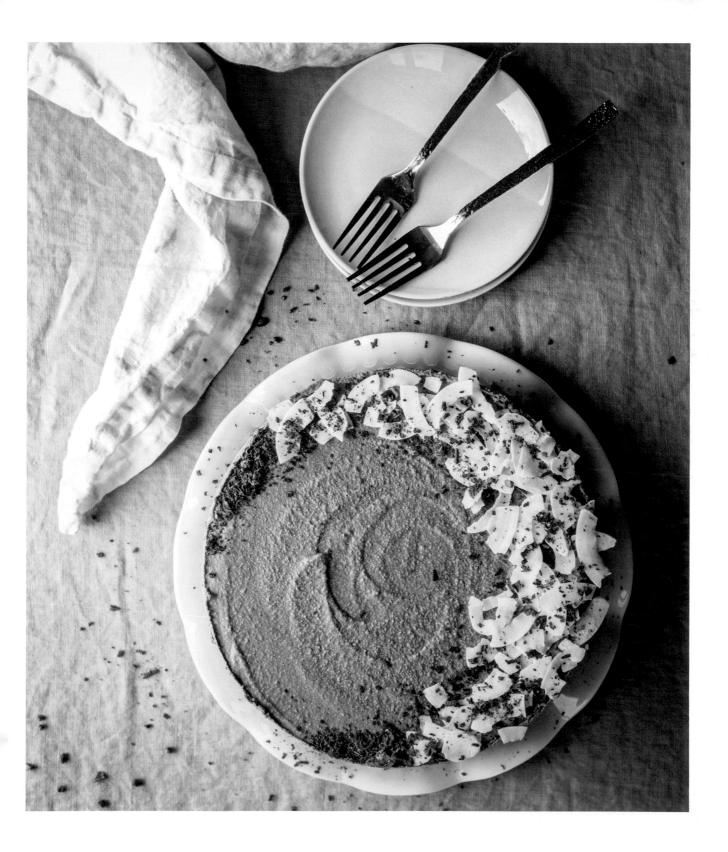

ABOUT THE AUTHOR

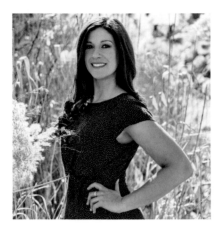

SAMANTHA GLADISH is a registered holistic nutritionist, metabolic balance weight loss coach and hormone fixer-upper. She is the founder of HolisticWellness.ca, a website dedicated to helping women lose weight and balance their hormones with delicious food. Samantha coaches and supports women from around the world on natural beauty care, holistic health and nutrition. Her philosophy is that through changing the way we eat, think, move and care for our bodies, we can heal ourselves and live a life of more power and possibility. Her passion for business is an extension of her work as a health coach. Samantha speaks internationally on all things health, wellness and entrepreneurship, and in her spare time, you can find her baking up delicious health-ified treats in her kitchen.

WORK WITH ME

Are you ready to dive in further and get a protocol and plan that is designed specifically for you? My team and I work online, coaching women globally and helping them get to the bottom of their hormone imbalances and weight gain. We provide customized protocols and plans, and we run lab work to further assess hormonal imbalances. Our treatment philosophy addresses optimizing nutrition, supplementation and lifestyle interventions.

VISIT ME: WWW.HOLISTICWELLNESS.CA

- Learn more about my Healthy Hormone Online Program: www.holisticwellness.ca/healthyhormones
- Tune into my Healthy Hormones for Women podcast: https://holisticwellness.ca/podcast

CONNECT WITH ME ON SOCIAL MEDIA:

- https://www.facebook.com/holisticwellnessfoodie
- https://instagram.com/holisticwellnessfoodie, @holisticwellnessfoodie
- https://twitter.com/IMHolistic

ACKNOWLEDGMENTS

Twenty-plus years of buying and reading books knowing that one day I'd be an author was a vision I held so dear to my heart, and I am so incredibly grateful for the love and support around me and to everyone who made this book journey possible. First off, thanks to Dr. Becky Campbell for connecting me with the amazing publishing team at Page Street Publishing. Becky—I am so grateful for your support, advice and direction.

Gaetan—my partner in life and in food! You are my biggest supporter and best friend. Thank you for always knowing how to hold space for me when I need it most and for always being a recipe-testing trouper.

Mom—for teaching me the importance of cooking from scratch. My love of food and cooking started with you, and I am so grateful for this incredible gift you have taught me.

Dad—for always letting me get whatever I wanted from the grocery store and for always being up to try one of my gluten-free desserts.

Nat Caron—thanks to your magical eye and seeing what I don't, you've always made every photoshoot come to life. It's a pleasure working with you every year.

Angela Doyon—thanks for always knowing exactly how to style my shoots and for creating a beautiful environment that is true to me and my brand.

Vanessa Fioretti—from content to design and running all things behind the scenes, you bring Holistic Wellness to life, and having you by my side makes everything that much easier and more fun. Thanks for designing the most beautiful infographics for this book!

Tina—I can always count on you to make me look beautiful, even in the wee early hours of the morning.

Trisha Hughes—I am honored that the recipes for my very first book got your incredible love and vision. The food photos in this book are beyond what I expected and I can't thank you enough for all that you do.

Nutrition Crew—Meghan, Joy, Julie and Marni, you inspire the heck outta me. Thank you for showing me what's possible and for always being open to sharing and offering insights.

The DeAngelis Family—who planted many "organic" seeds for me and Lily, for teaching me the most incredible way to cook artichokes. I am so grateful for your teachings, for opening your kitchen to me and for sharing insights about organic food, homeopathics and Chinese medicine. You all played a pivotal role in helping me connect to my true passion.

Page Street Publishing—to the kick-ass team that I've had the pleasure of working with over these last few months; I appreciate your listening to me, bringing my vision to life and trusting in me. Thank you to Karen, Meg, Marissa, Molly and Will.

Last and certainly not least, my Holistic Wellness community—for tuning in to my podcast, reading my blogs and posting and sharing your food photos on Instagram, you all inspire me so much and I am truly grateful for all your love and support.

REFERENCES

"Abhyanga: The Ayurvedic Daily Massage." Maharishi Ayurveda. https://www.mapi.com/ayurvedic-knowledge/massage/benefits-of-an-ayurvedic-abhyanga-massage.html.

"Adaptogens: Ancient Medicine for 21st Century Stress." Aviva Room. July 15, 2014. https://avivaromm.com/adaptogens-beating-stress.

"The Adrenal-Thyroid Connection." Amy Myers. March 2017. https://www.amymyersmd.com/2017/03/adrenal-thyroid-connection.

Alexander, L. M., and L. A. Straub-Bruce. Dental Herbalism: Natural Therapies for the Mouth. New York: Simon and Schuster, 2014.

"Are Saunas the Next Big Performance-Enhancing 'Drug'?" Dr. Joseph Mercola. May 24, 2014. https://articles.mercola.com/sites/articles/archive/2014/05/24/sauna-benefits.aspx.

Briden, L. Period Repair Manual. CreateSpace, 2018.

Brighten, J. Beyond the Pill: A 30-Day Program to Balance Your Hormones, Reclaim Your Body, and Reverse the Dangerous Side Effects of the Birth Control Pill. New York: HarperCollins, 2019.

Casagrande, S. S., C. C. Cowie, and J. E. Fradkin. "Utility of the US Preventive Services Task Force Criteria for Diabetes Screening." American Journal of Preventive Medicine 45, no. 2 (2013): 167–174.

Doheny, K. "Birth Control Pills, HRT Tied to Digestive Ills." Health Day, May 21, 2012.

"Drugs in Our Drinking Water?" WebMD/Kathleen Doheny. March 10, 2008. https://www.webmd.com/a-to-z-guides/features/drugs-in-our-drinking-water#1.

Eisenstein, M. "Digestive Issues." Nutrition Digest 38, no. 2 (original publication: NOHA NEWS, Summer 2007). http://americannutritionassociation.org/newsletter/digestive-issues.

"Estrogen Metabolism." Revolution Health & Wellness. https://www.revolutionhealth.org/estrogen-metabolism.

Evert, A. B., J. L. Boucher, M. Cypress, S. A. Dunbar, M. J. Franz, E. J. Mayer-Davis, J. J. Neumiller, et al. "Nutrition Therapy Recommendations for the Management of Adults with Diabetes." Diabetes Care 37, supplement 1 (2014): S120–S143.

Fasano, A., and T. Shea-Donohue. "Mechanisms of Disease: The Role of Intestinal Barrier Function in the Pathogenesis of Gastrointestinal Autoimmune Diseases." Nature Clinical Practice Gastroenterology & Hepatology 2, no. 9 (2005): 416–422.

Franz, M. J., J. L. Boucher, and A. B. Evert. "Evidence-Based Diabetes Nutrition Therapy Recommendations Are Effective: The Key Is Individualization." Diabetes, Metabolic Syndrome and Obesity: Targets and Therapy 7 (2014): 65.

Fröhlich, M., A. Döring, A. Imhof, W. L. Hutchinson, M. B. Pepys, and W. Koenig. "Oral Contraceptive Use Is Associated with a Systemic Acute Phase Response." Fibrinolysis and Proteolysis 13, no. 6 (1999): 239–244.

Funfack, W. Metabolic Balance®—Nutrition Basics: Introduction to the Success Program. Südwest Verlag, 2011.

Galletta, M., S. Grasso, A. Vaiarelli, and S. J. Roseff. "Bye-bye Chiro-inositol-myo-inositol: True Progress in the Treatment of Polycystic Ovary Syndrome and Ovulation Induction." European Review for Medical Pharmacological Sciences 15, no. 10 (2011): 1212–1214.

Hickman, R. J., T. Khambaty, and J. C. Stewart. "C-reactive Protein Is Elevated in Atypical but Not Nonatypical Depression: Data from the National Health and Nutrition Examination Survey (NHANES) 1999–2004." Journal of Behavioral Medicine 37, no. 4 (2014): 621–629.

"The Inflammation from A1 Milk Is Mind-Boggling." Lara Briden. February 20, 2013. https://www.larabriden.com/the-inflammation-from-a1-milk-is-mind-boggling.

Keller, U. "Dietary Proteins in Obesity and in Diabetes." International Journal for Vitamin and Nutrition Research 81, no. 2 (2011): 125.

Khan, S. H., A. Ijaz, S. A. Bokhari, M. S. Hanif, and N. Azam. "Frequency of Impaired Glucose Tolerance and Diabetes Mellitus in Subjects with Fasting Blood Glucose Below 6.1 mmol/L [110 mg/dL]." Eastern Mediterranean Health Journal 19, no. 2 (2013): 175–180.

Maxwell, C., and S. L. Volpe. "Effect of Zinc Supplementation on Thyroid Hormone Function." Annals of Nutrition and Metabolism 51, no. 2 (2007): 188–194.

Mu, Q., J. Kirby, C. M. Reilly, and X. M. Luo. "Leaky Gut as a Danger Signal for Autoimmune Diseases." Frontiers in Immunology 8 (2017): 598.

Nordio, M., and S. Basciani. "Treatment with Myo-inositol and Selenium Ensures Euthyroidism in Patients with Autoimmune Thyroiditis." International Journal of Endocrinology (2017). https://doi.org/10.1155/2017/2549491.

Nordio, M., and R. Pajalich. "Combined Treatment with Myo-inositol and Selenium Ensures Euthyroidism in Subclinical Hypothyroidism Patients with Autoimmune Thyroiditis." Journal of Thyroid Research (2013). https://doi.org/10.1155/2013/424163.

Nordio, M., and E. Proietti. "The Combined Therapy with Myo-inositol and D-chiro-inositol Reduces the Risk of Metabolic Disease in PCOS Overweight Patients Compared to Myo-inositol Supplementation Alone." European Review of Medical Pharmacological Sciences 16, no. 5 (2012): 575–581.

"Normal Blood Sugar Levels for Adults with Diabetes." WebMD. January 25, 2018. http://www.webmd.com/diabetes/guide/normal-blood-sugar-levels-chart-adults.

Panda, S., and A. Kar. "Changes in Thyroid Hormone Concentrations after Administration of Ashwagandha Root Extract to Adult Male Mice." *Journal of Pharmacy and Pharmacology* 50, no. 9 (1998): 1065–1068.

Pase, M. P., J. J. Himali, A. S. Beiser, H. J. Aparicio, C. L. Satizabal, R. S. Vasan, S. Seshadri, and P. F. Jacques. "Sugar and Artificially Sweetened Beverages and the Risks of Incident Stroke and Dementia: A Prospective Cohort Study." *Stroke* 48, no. 5 (2017): 1139–1146.

"Powerful and Simple Tips to Help Lower Your EMF Risks," Dr. Joseph Mercola. February 9, 2011. https://articles.mercola.com/sites/articles/archive/2011/02/09/powerful-and-simple-tips-to-help-lower-your-emf-risks.aspx.

"RHR: Is a Disrupted Gut Microbiome at the Root of Modern Disease?—with Dr. Justin Sonnenburg." Chris Kresser. March 16, 2019. https://chriskresser.com/is-a-disrupted-gut-microbiome-at-the-root-of-modern-disease-with-dr-justin-sonnenburg.

"Six Essential Supplements for Your Thyroid and Hashimoto's." Aviva Romm. May 16, 2018. https://avivaromm.com/essential-thyroid-supplements.

Tirosh, A., I. Shai, D. Tekes-Manova, E. Israeli, D. Pereg, T. Shochat, I. Kochba, and A. Rudich. "Normal Fasting Plasma Glucose Levels and Type 2 Diabetes in Young Men." *New England Journal of Medicine* 353, no. 14 (2005): 1454–1462.

"Treating the Gut Is Vitally Important for Autism Spectrum Disorders." Nicole Beurkens. April 17, 2018. https://www.drbeurkens.com/gut-treatment-for-autism-spectrum-disorders.

Visser, J., J. Rozing, A. Sapone, K. Lammers, and A. Fasano. "Tight Junctions, Intestinal Permeability, and Autoimmunity: Celiac Disease and Type 1 Diabetes Paradigms." *Annals of the New York Academy of Sciences* 1165, no. 1 (2009): 195–205.

Won, E., and Y. K. Kim. "Stress, the Autonomic Nervous System, and the Immune-kynurenine Pathway in the Etiology of Depression." *Current Neuropharmacology* 14, no. 7 (2016): 665–673.

RESOURCES

Here is a list of products and brands I have trusted and used over the years myself and with my clients.

SUPPLEMENTS

- Activation Products
- Anima Mundi Herbals
- AOR (Advanced Orthomolecular Research)
- CanPrev
- Cyto-Matrix
- Designs for Health
- Genestra
- Genuine Health
- Martin & Pleasance
- Moodbeli
- Natural Calm
- NFH
- NOW Foods
- Organic Traditions
- Pascoe
- Perfect Keto
- Pure Encapsulations
- PURICA
- St. Francis Herb Farm
- Vital Proteins

FOOD

- Acropolis Organics olive oil and balsamic vinegar
- Bob's Red Mill
- Enjoy Life chocolate chips
- Four Sigmatic
- Lily's Sweets chocolate
- Navitas Organics
- NOW Foods
- Nuts To You Nut Butters
- Organic Traditions superfoods and snacks
- Primal Kitchen
- Primal Palate
- Redmond Real Salt
- Simply Organic

TEAS AND COFFEE

- Bulletproof Coffee
- Flora
- Four Sigmatic
- Herbaria
- Traditional Medicinals
- Yogi tea

ONLINE HEALTH SHOPS

- Natura Market
- Pure Feast
- Thrive Market

CLEAN BEAUTY: SKIN CARE AND MAKEUP

- Annmarie Gianni Skin Care
- Beautycounter
- Consonant Skincare
- Inika Organic
- Living Libations
- Raww Cosmetics
- RMS Beauty
- Sukin
- W3LL PEOPLE
- 100% Pure

INDEX